for Elda Hartley

Christmas 1988

from

Gene Kieffer

D0869504

Gopi Krishna

Higher

Consciousness

The Evolutionary

Thrust of Kundalini

Published by:
F.I.N.D. Research Trust
and
Kundalini Research Foundation, Ltd.

Higher Consciousness

First printing 1974

Second printing 1988

Published by:

F.I.N.D. Research Trust
R.R. 5 Flesherton
Ontario, Canada
N0C 1E0

The Kundalini Research Foundation, Ltd.
P.O. Box 2248
Noroton Heights
CT. 06820
U.S.A.

Published in association with:

Kundalini Research Association International

Kundalini Research and Publication Trust
D-291 Sarvodaya Enclave
New Delhi 110017, India

Kundalini Research Association
Gemsenstrasse 7,
8006 Zurich, Switzerland

Bioenergy Research Foundation
1187 Coast Village Road, 1-186 Santa Barbara
CA. 93108., U.S.A.

First F.I.N.D. Research Trust edition

First Kundalini Research Foundation, Ltd. edition

International Standards Book Number:
087097-061-5

Library of Congress Catalog Card Number:
74-75418

Contents

3   Religion and Evolution

4   Yoga and Higher Consciousness

Introduction

Any book by Pandit Gopi Krishna is a very special event.

He is unique among writers on the subject of higher consciousness because what he has to say is from *his own direct experience.* This fact is still too novel for the general public to realize the staggering implications.

In a modern world in which trendy "transcendentalism" through drugs or meditation techniques is a commodity exploited by self-appointed Gurus for their own vanity, when new cults spring up over-night with millions of followers attracted through publicity in the mass media or the self-deception of crowds rather than true spiritual insight, Gopi Krishna has been virtually a lone voice in the tradition of the great sages and seers of ancient India.

He never sought to establish new cults or a mass following, being a humble, absolutely sincere, and modest man. He was dedicated only to revealing the special insights gained by his own mystical experience of higher consciousness, the genuine transcendental state described by Yogis and saints thousands of years ago, an experience that has become legendary in modern times.

In his earlier book, *Kundalini: The Evolutionary Energy in Man* (1967; 1970), Gopi Krishna described how he aroused the mysterious *kundalini* force, that secret power-reservoir in the human body, and achieved that mystical experience of higher consciousness that had become so rare as to be fabulous:

"Suddenly, with a roar like that of a waterfall, I felt a stream of liquid light entering my brain through the spinal cord....I felt the point of consciousness that was myself growing wider, surrounded by waves of light...."

This sudden awakening of the secret *kundalini* force came about through the practice of Yoga, but he was not prepared for its fantastic onset. It endangered his health and even his life for many years, until he learned to live with it, modify its effects, and cooperate with the biological changes it brought about in his brain and body.

He writes, therefore, with absolute authority; and it is important for a modern world, bewildered by a breakdown in true values, to read and consider carefully all that he has to say. For here are genuine insights *arising from an actual condition of higher consciousness.* They are not the theories, wishful thinking, or rehashes of those who have never had such an experience. The condition of higher consciousness is so rare and truly transcendental that mankind cannot afford to ignore any single instance in modern times. We are privileged in being able to consider and verify its revelations from an individual in our time rather than from the records of the past in sacred scriptures.

Can one really believe this, in a world of false claims and charlatans? I can affirm that I *know* it to be true. I have always taken a special interest in the phenomenon of *kundalini* and have met several individuals in whom this extraordinary power has been aroused in some degree. I knew Gopi Krishna personally and had inspiring conversations with him in India. His work has been supported by eminent scientists, and a Kundalini Research Foundation has been established. I can confirm his absolute genuineness and sincerity.

He writes with a refreshing and touching humility. He never concealed his wonder that destiny should have granted him this awakening into higher consciousness. He stressed that this experience, so immeasurably more profound and inspiring than normal consciousness and absolutely blissful in nature, is yet only a hint of still higher states. And he knew only too well that the immensities of consciousness and perception are sometimes too much for the mental and physical apparatus that tries to convey them in the inadequate medium of words in a printed book.

He had no special advantages of birth or education. In his great inspiration the words tumbled out at speed, and sometimes the command of a language not his own was inadequate to express the marvelous vistas of life and human destiny that opened to his vision like a blaze of dazzling light. For he perceived always with full waking consciousness, unlike the passive trance of the spiritualist medium or the stupor of the drugtaker.

Some of his new awareness is so inconceivable to the consciousness of ordinary individuals that it is remarkable that he could find words to express himself at all. It is a situation rather like that of a great author forced to type at speed on an old and imperfect typewriter with a foreign keyboard! When the experience of Cosmic Consciousness or Superconsciousness becomes accessible to other individuals, as Gopi Krishna believed could happen soon, there will be many different accounts to confirm such insights. And it may be that great writers, poets, musicians, and scientists will be inspired to supplement these visions with all the eloquence and art with which they are already gifted.

Do not be put off by the unfamiliarity of terms like *kundalini*. There is unfortunately no real modern equivalent to this ancient Hindu science of the soul. Although originally surrounded with mythological concepts of the union of a god and goddess in terms of a complex Hindu metaphysical doctrine, it is now clear that there is a real biological basis for this extraordinary power center of latent energy within the human body and in the cosmos as a whole. This force is located at the base of the human spine, nourished by energy from food, air, ethical and spiritual development. It can be expressed in sexual activity or transmuted into a subtle form that rises up the spinal column to a center in the brain, enlarging the consciousness. The sudden spiral movement from the base of the spine has been called "The Serpent Power" by the ancients, and mythological forms of this basic fact have been elaborated into stories of a man, a woman, a serpent and the tree of knowledge in a primal garden, common to many different religions.

This force is evolutionary, both in its expression of the procreative urge and its internal union within the human body, opening the door to the inspired consciousness that guides the progress of the human race through sages, seers, geniuses, and artists. This force is slowly modifying human biological structure through vital currents in the body. For a fuller understanding of these bare facts, it is essential to study other books by Gopi Krishna. In the present one, using straightforward questions and answers, he discusses some of the implications for both religion and science.

Out of his own experience, which remained with him in a never-ending meditation, he has a message for each individual reader that he or she may personally weigh the meaning of this primary phenomenon, its connections with great spiritual teachings, and its incredible evolutionary role in the destiny of all life and consciousness. Gopi Krishna shows how we can understand and cooperate with this force and live in harmony with its purpose, confirming what religious and ethical leaders have always taught: There has to be creative change within each individual, based on individual efforts, refining understanding of one's place in the scheme of life.

If this seems at first less sensational than the shortcuts promised by modern pop Gurus, that is only a deceptive initial impression. Gopi Krishna enlarges on the meaning of total life and the contribution that will be made by a reformed religion and open-minded science, in a future destiny of the human race beyond the wildest dreams of modern thinkers.

This book speaks directly to your own judgment. It makes no imperious demands and does not demand to be taken on trust. In a world of the spurious, catchpenny, dishonest, and power-seeking, there is an incredible satisfaction in contacting once again simple truth which can guide us through modern perplexities.

During his lifetime, Gopi Krishna had a special message for scientists and scholars. He pleaded for experiments to validate the reality of the arousal of *kundalini* and its biological effects in the human organism. He offered cooperation in investigating scientific aspects of his own condition — a living example of a development so rare that we are fortunate in having such an individual in our own lifetime.

It is sad to record that he is no longer with us in person. He passed away in July 1984 at the good age of 81, but happily he has left us a score of books and tape recordings to keep alive his vital message to humanity.

The present book gives clear guidance to the great questions of meaning and purpose in life in a simple question and answer format.

I urge every individual to study this book with honesty and sincerity, and experience the joy of self-discovery; to develop awareness of the greatest enigma of human experience — the meaning of life itself.

Leslie Shepard

1 The Physical Aspects of Higher Consciousness

■ For many centuries, the attainment of a higher state of consciousness has been the goal of mystics of many religions in order to resolve the age-old riddle of man's relationship to his creator. Yoga teachings have stressed the concept of kundalini—The Serpent Power—and have taught that it is a dormant energy that may be aroused by certain disciplines and result in transcendental awareness. What do terms like "transcendental" and "higher consciousness" mean and what should be the characteristics of one who has attained to a higher state of consciousness?

Attainment of a higher level of consciousness implies overstepping the boundaries of the human state. Anyone who claims to have gained transcendental awareness or approach to Divinity must, in some respects, have exceeded the normal limits of the human mind and experience.

It is necessary that such an enlightened person be pious and righteous, free from ego, desire, attachment, hate, envy, aggression, violence, lust, and other unholy traits, of course, but these things are not in themselves the criteria of higher consciousness. People are naturally constituted in different ways, some having inherently less lust, passion, avarice, aggression and more of the nobler attributes, while others have more of the animal characteristics. The normal range of human beings includes men with saintly character at one end of the scale and virtual devils, criminals, and murderers at the other. In none of these cases is the human limit exceeded.

There are some people who are so saintly in character that it appears impossible for a normal man to emulate them. At the same time there are evil-doers whose hideous deeds strike terror into the hearts of others. We encounter both of these extremes in everyday life. But a saintly person, with all his piety and holiness, may not show any remarkable intellectual superiority as compared to a normal intelligent individual, while at the other end of the scale some criminals show such extraordinary talent for crime that one is amazed at their wit and resourcefulness. Therefore, unless there are certain marked characteristics distinguishing an individual claiming a higher state of consciousness from the other average or even extraordinary individuals, we can only treat such a person as belonging to the normal category.

If the reality of spiritual experience and the possibility of a higher state of consciousness are to be convincingly demonstrated, there must be incontrovertible evidence to show that an enlightened man or woman can develop a mental stature that is entirely beyond the reach of normal individuals, however intelligent or talented they might be. If this evidence is not forthcoming, there has been no overstepping of the human traits.

"The knower of Brahman attains the highest," says the Taittriya Upanishad (II. i.). "Brahman is truth, knowledge and infinity. He who knows that Brahman, as existing in the intellect, lodged in the supreme space in the head, enjoys, as identified with the all-knowing Brahman, all desirable things simultaneously."

According to Shankaracharya, a highly developed personality is needed even in one who aspires to the Supreme State: "The truth of the Paramatman is extremely subtle and cannot be reached by the gross outgoing tendency of the mind." In Vivekachudamani (361), he also says; "It is only accessible to noble souls with perfectly pure minds, by means of Samādhi [meditative trance] brought on by an extraordinary fineness of the mental state."

■ *There are some Yogis who can reduce their breathing to such an extent that it becomes almost imperceptible. Some can arrest the flow of blood or diminish the rhythm of the heart to such a degree that their bodies assume a corpselike condition, and in this state can be buried underground or interred in hermetically sealed boxes for many days without succumbing to death. On being exhumed they revive as if they had been asleep all the while. Isn't this a feat entirely beyond the capacity of a normal individual to perform?*

The superiority of the enlightened person does not lie in bizarre physical demonstrations, but in the development of a transhuman consciousness and rapport with the Cosmic Intelligence and invisible conscious forces not perceptible to normal people. The tendency to hibernate is present in bears, frogs, and other creatures and does not carry with it any enhancement of consciousness. The attempt to duplicate the performance of these lowly creatures can only be regarded as regressive rather than progressive, for enlightened consciousness cannot proceed from artificially distorted or arrested functions of the body, but rather from a harmonious working of the metabolic processes and bodily rhythms.

A classical example of suspended animation was provided by Haridass, a Hatha-Yogi, in the time of Maharaja Ranjit Singh in 1873. Under the orders of the Maharaja, the Yogi entered into a trance and in that condition was shut in a wooden box four feet by three. The Maharaja sealed the lock, and the box was placed in a cellar also similarly locked and sealed. A strict watch was maintained over the building for a period of forty days. Every precaution was taken to eliminate fraud. At the end of the period, Sir Claude Wade, British Resident in the Maharaja's court, and a medical doctor, together with the Maharaja and others, had the seals broken and the body lifted out of the box. Medical examination revealed that there was no pulse at the wrist or temples and no sounds from the heart, only a little warmth at the top of the head. The Yogi's disciples massaged his body with clarified butter and hot water and put his tongue, which had been drawn backward in the position called Khechari Mudra, into the natural position.

After a while, Haridass returned to life. The account of this extraordinary feat was given by Sir Claude and a German physician who was with the Maharaja at the time. Haridass repeated his performance several times. And the feat has been duplicated by other Hatha-Yogis since then. A distinguishing feature in the performance of Haridass is that it was very well authenticated.

Another similar incident occurred in Hardwar, India, in the second decade of this century. The Yogi, when asked about his condition during the internment for a period lasting several weeks, said that he remembered nothing. This is a common state of mind of those who practice advanced *pranayama* or Yogic breathing techniques, with consequent arrest of the metabolic processes. The condition is called Jada-Samādhi. "Jada" means insentient.

Apart from his remarkable suspension of normal physical functions, Haridass showed no evidence of any spiritual qualities. It is even said that he lacked higher ethical development. Today there are still Yogis in India who can stop their breathing or heart action for considerable periods, or they can perform

other extraordinary bodily feats for the sake of gain or simply to
show off their talents. There is no doubt in the case of born
mystics, mediums, and other sensitives, however, that a trance-
like condition, often with diminished breathing and heart
action, can supervene at the time of ecstasy or psychic manifestations; but this is far removed from the state of suspended animation of the Hatha-Yogi.

Experiments with the well-known drug marijuana have shown
that when injected in a pure form in dogs it can induce a state
of suspended animation up to eight days, after which the animal
returns to normal functioning. Further experiments are in progress to utilize this hibernation property of the drug on battle-
fields, to put an injured soldier into a state of suspended
animation until medical aid becomes available. In the light of
this discovery it is easy to infer that, as the result of extreme
forms of *pranayama*, the chemical reactions caused in some
people can induce hiberation for varying periods of time. Hence
those who place reliance on such external symptoms for corroboration of the transcendent states of consciousness induced
by Yoga can easily see the falsity of their position.

The Hatha-Yoga ascetics who go to this extreme clearly display the same fanaticism that characterizes the Urdhavabahus
who keep one or both arms raised until they become inflexibly
withered, or the Akashamukhins, who keep their necks bent
back, gazing at the sky until this attitude becomes habitual and
the neck becomes fixed in this position. These are not means to
salvation but remnants of austerities and penances of primitive
society. Mutilations, biting of the scalp, severe beating, knocking
out teeth, fasting, chopping off lumps of flesh, exposure to the
bites of virulent ants, and other such self-inflicted tortures were
a common feature of tribal life in North and South America,
Africa, and Australia at the time of adolescence in boys and girls
in the ritual ordeals of crude religious beliefs.

It is unfortunate that the main armory of research on Yoga and allied spiritual disciplines should have centered around breathing and pulse rates of the practitioners, in order to seek physiological corroboration of the extraordinary states of consciousness supposed to be associated with them. Is there any historical record to show that great spiritual prodigies of antiquity like Buddha, Jesus Christ, or the seers of the Upanishads, or the mystics of more recent times, had a malfunctioning metabolic system, or that it was with a diminished pulse and heart action that they performed their prodigious feats of conversion or produced their outstanding inspired scriptures and teachings? What error in thinking is driving earnest seekers and other honest investigators to devote their time and energy to an exploration based on the mistaken view that transcendental states of consciousness are invariably attended by diminished or altered metabolic processes?

There are certainly other physiological symptoms present in the enlightened by which the validity of spiritual experience can be empirically established and determined. The most prominent of these is Urdhava-retas, or the upward streaming of the reproductive energy in the awakened individual. This fact has been known in India for at least four thousand years and is symbolically represented in every temple and shrine in which *lingam* or *lingam* and *yoni*, as creative symbols, are housed for adoration. They are to remind the worshippers that the same life-energy that, as the fruit of parental conjugation, becomes the cause of our birth is also designed by nature to effect our release from the bonds of the flesh when it rises to the *brahmarandra* in the brain, uniting with the conscious principle and setting it free from the otherwise inescapable prison house of the phenomenal world. It is this life-energy, the source behind propagation and evolution both, which is called *kundalini* and from ancient times has been regarded as a goddess.

The upward flow of the reproductive energy is to be understood in its natural form as an altered activity of the cerebrospinal system and the organs of generation. The methods to effect this activity recommended in some books on Hatha-Yoga are revolting in the extreme. An example is the practice of Vajroli Mudra, in which a thin metal tube is inserted through the urethra and liquids of progressive density absorbed and discharged in the initial stages. The practice is designed to develop absolute control over the seminal fluid, its emission and reabsorption. The statements on sexual techniques in the ancient manuals on Hatha-Yoga, such as the Goraksha Samhita (61–71) and the Hathayoga Pradipika (III–82), referred to by Dr. Mircea Eliade in his book, Yoga, Immortality and Freedom, are, therefore, to be viewed with caution.

The arousal of *kundalini* is not designed by nature as a means for sexual gratification in this artificial way, but to create a new physiological activity in the body in which the upward flow of the energy occurs spontaneously and becomes a natural biological function of the organism. In fact, as is generally held, the sublimination of sexual energy usually occurs to an appreciable degree in the case of men of genius, great intellectuals, poets, painters, musicians, and the like.

■ *If there is an evolutionary process at work in the human organism, why has it not been understood and detected a long time ago? Why is it so difficult to locate? What is the aim of this evolutionary impulse, and do those who succeed in awakening this power become all-wise?*

The mechanism has not been understood in modern times because the physiological reactions of awakened *kundalini*, although observed by the ancients, have not yet been investigated or interpreted in the light of present-day knowledge of the human body. In view of the tremendous developments in our knowledge of the physical universe during recent years, it is of the utmost importance that those interested in human welfare should take a new look at all the spiritual doctrines, systems, and ideas of the past.

In my earlier books, I have tried to make it clear that the religious impulse is only an expression of the evolutionary urge in human beings, and that there is already present in the biological structure of man an inherent natural tendency to reach an expanded state of consciousness. In order to achieve this natural, predetermined target, every human body, from birth to death, is in a state of perennial internal activity, resulting from processes that ebb and flow, to adjust the whole system to a new form of awareness not possible with the existing psychosomatic structure of the organism. In spite of the current prodigious increase in knowledge of the human body, this activity of the evolutionary mechanism is still completely unknown.

There is no doubt that competent investigation, directed toward Yoga and other religious phenomena, will ultimately lead to an understanding of the mechanism, as also of the details of processes that are imperceptibly but ceaselessly at work in the human body to mold the cerebrospinal system to a higher state of perception in which consciousness becomes the predominant reality of the universe. These processes are not easily detectable by the methods at present employed by science, but they may become discernible in the near future.

We observe the process of growth in a child clearly with our own eyes. We see how a growing infant, moving its arms and kicking its legs in the cradle, learns of its own accord to turn from side to side, and from lying flat on its back, by a change of position, to crawl on the floor. Then it begins to toddle, and when proficient in this makes repeated attempts, at first abortive and later successful, to stand erect. After this achievement it tries to walk, often falling in the initial stages, but rising up again immediately, continues the exercise until it becomes habitual. In the same way, from the repetition of mere babbling sounds it learns to talk and finally develops into a fully formed human being.

We can study all these stages of development in the minutest detail, watch every movement of the muscles, the tongue and lips, witness the accelerated metabolism, the rapid pulse and rate of respiration, enhanced digestive and eliminatory processes, mark the increasing stature and the growing size of the body, but we are as yet unable to know what transpires in the child's brain and nervous system to regulate and channelize this complex process of growth unerringly in a certain predetermined direction. Here we stand defeated before the still unfathomed mystery of life.

If this is our position with regard to a common biological process that occurs before our very eyes, how can we expect that we should at once reach to the very roots of the process of transformation generated by an awakened *kundalini*? Furthermore, cases of awakening are extremely rare and the whole phenomenon has, from the very beginning, been wrapped in such a cloak of mystery and superstition that before attempting to investigate the biological processes responsible, it is necessary to establish the actual existence of the mechanism and the possibility of transformation of consciousness. When this has been done, the real research will follow as a matter of course.

Even intelligent people can be naive in this matter. When they come to know of an individual who claims to have won to a transhuman state of consciousness, they often conclude that he has instantly become an all-knowing entity or a walking encyclopedia. They forget that it has taken the labor of millions and a time span of millennia for knowledge of the physical world to grow to its present capacity. How then can spiritual knowledge take such a prodigious leap that one who has gained the first rung of the ladder of spiritual illumination should be able to reveal all the hidden mysteries of the cosmos? The harvest of this false belief can be seen in the lavish and fantastic accounts of the superconscious world in the voluminous works of many of those credited with higher states of consciousness.

It is not in the performance of amazing physical feats or in the working of miracles or in encyclopedic knowledge that the value of expanded consciousness lies. There can be no more amazing feats than have already been achieved by mankind with the proper use of intellect. The crown of superconsciousness is designed by heaven to enable mortals ultimately to realize their own imperishable nature and to win access to the shoreless ocean of Cosmic Intelligence.

During the course of this tremendous evolutionary development, of which the birth of civilization marks only the completion of the first stage, the more highly evolved individuals in the various spheres of human knowledge and art, by an inherent tendency of gifted men to make their talents widely known, help to raise the less evolved to their own height. When this transition is complete the earth will be a paradise and mankind will enter upon a golden age that has no parallel in previous history.

Apart from references to the arousal of *kundalini* in ancient documents and modern writings on the subject, there has been no objective demonstration of the phenomenon in recent times. The instances cited by Dr. Vincent Rele in his *The Mysterious Kundalini* (Bombay, 1927), do not at all represent a case of transformed consciousness. The fact that someone can swallow poison and perform other startling feats is no guarantee that he has an awakened *kundalini*. Arrest of the flow of blood in the arm or leg or any other part of the body, diminution of the pulse or suspension of respiration can be achieved with long practice by determined individuals with a certain degree of command over their autonomic nervous system. Performances of this nature appear amazing because they are so difficult to duplicate, but the human organism has tremendous potentialities and possibilities, which are demonstrated every day in the hazardous feats of mountain climbers, athletes, circus performers, deep-sea divers, and the like. The linkage of diminished breathing and pulse rate, arrested flow of blood, coldness or cataleptic condition of the body, with the awakening of *kundalini* has been a cause of great misunderstanding and has led to erroneous notions about this power.

■ *Can the psychosomatic mechanism of* kundalini *be demonstrated to the satisfaction of science?*

As far as my experience goes, I believe that a scientific demonstration of this psychophysiological mechanism is possible with the methods already known to science. Had the arousal of this force no perceptible effects on the human body, the ancient masters would not have devoted their attention to the enumeration of various signs and symptoms that occur on the awakening. They would not have made repeated mention of the phenomenon of lights that attend the arousal or have meticulously described the nature of the sounds heard, likening them to thunder, humming of bees, roaring of waterfalls, or the pealing of bells; and the lights to the luster of the moon, the radiance of the sun, the dazzling flash of lightning, or the glow of fire. Nor would they have been able to furnish precise descriptions of the *cakras* (nerve clusters) and specify their particular locations on the cerebrospinal axis. In fact, the ancient authors have taken considerable pains to pinpoint the exact location of the *kanda*, the inverted triangle below the navel on which *kundalini* rests.

Their descriptions leave no doubt that it is the region intimately connected with the reproductive organs and that it functions as the powerhouse for generating the life currents that lead to expanded states of consciousness.

Even a cursory glance at the descriptions contained in ancient texts make it clear that the authors have spared no effort to explain the physiological implications of their researches. The *cakras*, generally accepted to be seven in number, are all situated at vital spots in the body, commanding the organs of reproduction, elimination, digestion, blood circulation, respiration, ideation, and the modalities of consciousness. *Kundalini*, it is said, pierces all these *cakras* before entering the *sahasrara*, or the seventh center in the brain. These statements confirm to the student of physiology that after arousal, the energy released by *kundalini* circulates in all the vital organs, including the brain. The descriptions of the hypothetical lotuses and *shaktis* or goddesses are easy to understand in the light of the religious beliefs and elementary knowledge of human physiology at the time. But we can be sure about the basic fact that these descriptions are intended to signify the involvement of all the important organs of the body in the process of transformation set in motion by this divine energy.

The meticulous descriptions of the *nadis* and the stress on their number provides further evidence that the ancient masters referred to the carriers of impulses and sensations in the body—in other words, to the nerves. The statement that there are thousands of *nadis*, fine like a spider's thread or the hairy fiber of a lotus stalk, is a clear indication that they are the nerves made of flesh and not any imaginary astral conduits. Again, the localization of the channels—called *ida, pingala,* and *sushumna*—on either side or through the center of the spinal cord, from its base to the point of termination, can only signify that the cerebrospinal axis is ultimately connected with the process of awaken-

ing regenerative impulses and that they cause an alteration in
the state of consciousness. There is no reason for putting a different interpretation on the unambiguous statements of the
ancient writers by carrying the whole phenomenon of *kundalini*
into unverifiable metaphysical realms. It should be treated as a
psychophysiological operation of the body, understandable in
the context of known physiological laws and verifiable by science.

The main difficulty in presenting the phenomenon of *kundalini* to the general public, as a legitimate function of the human
organism to enhance the capacity of the brain, lies in the fact
that both the traditional concepts and the modern versions of
the ancient writings treat it as a divine dispensation, uncon-
nected with the biological structure of the body. There is a
tendency among some modern writers to dwell more on the
miraculous and the supernatural aspects of the phenomenon
than on its physiological background. The habit of ancient
authors to ascribe supernatural causes to every occurrence not
easily explainable by the intellect should not cloud the judgment
of the writers who try to interpret their works today. If the
present practice of uncritical acceptance of such attitudes continues, the true doctrine of *kundalini* will never see the light of
reason. On the contrary, it will become more complex and
obscure as fresh groups of commentators try to penetrate deeper
into the cryptic meanings and intricacies of the terms used by
the ancient masters.

In the old books, there is generally an undue emphasis on
mantras (ritualistic incantations), *siddhis* (psychic powers) and
all the highly embellished metaphysical jargon, both relevant
and irrelevant. From a study of these works one might infer
that the authors believed in the possibility of a miraculous
change in human consciousness without in the least affecting
the body or the brain. Such a conclusion is unrealistic. We are
all aware of the hard and fast limits imposed by the brain on the

state of individual consciousness. A whole range of imperfect expressions of intelligence confronts us in the case of Mongoloids, cretins, imbeciles, idiots, and other categories of imperfectly developed individuals. Has it ever been possible, or can anyone now make it possible, to raise the consciousness of one of these unfortunates even to the level of ordinary people? If not, how can we even think of raising the consciousness of an average person to divine proportions without first regenerating the brain?

If the awakening of *kundalini* merely represents the operation of a divine cosmic energy, acting through invisible astral channels to bestow the boon of Cosmic Consciousness on a devotee, then one deficient in intelligence can be as good a recipient of grace as an exceptional man. Even the ancient writers realized the impossibility of such a transformation. This is the reason why they insisted on certain mental and physical attributes.

The distinguishing characteristics of promising aspirants are meticulously described not only in books on Raja-Yoga but also in the Tantras and in treatises on Hatha-Yoga. "A deliberative mind is the Mantra," says Shivasutra (2. 1). According to Mundaka Upanishad (III i. 8), "It [the Self] is not comprehended through eye, nor through speech, nor through the other senses, nor is it attained through austerity or Karma [actions]. Only when one becomes purified in mind through the blessings of a discerning intellect can he then see that indivisible Self through meditation."

Discussing the nature of the intellect indispensable for enlightenment, the Bhagavad-Gita says (18. 30), "That which knoweth energy and abstinence, what ought to be done and what ought not to be done, fear and fearlessness, bondage and liberation, that Buddhi (intellect) is pure, O Partha." A discriminating and pure intellect is necessary in those born for a divine state, according to the Gita and other scriptures of India. "Aloof from

misery, contented, without conflict, free from jealousy, given to
the knowledge of doctrine, peaceful," says the Kularnava Tantra
LX-84, 85), "without insolence, anger, show, desire and ego,
truthful in speech, not fickle."

Again (XI-98): "The mainspring of Kula-dharma lies not in
elaborate rituals, like Abhiseka, not in Mantra, not in poring
over learned treatises, but in a truthful ordering of life." All
Indian scriptures, all the authoritative treatises dealing with
Yoga, invariably prescribe noble attributes of mind, surrender to
Divine Will, truthfulness, compassion, selflessness, and other
virtues as the prerequisites for the attainment of higher states of
consciousness. The body and the mind have to be purified by
reasonable austerity and noble ways of thought and action.

"All the gods dwell in the body," says the Gupta-Diksha
Tantra, meaning thereby that the divine states ascribed to gods
reside in the body and may be experienced as the result of certain disciplines employed to make the body a suitable vehicle for
the purpose. It is obvious that the fundamental issue to be
resolved for a student of Yoga is the relationship between the
body and transcendental consciousness. To suppose that higher
states of consciousness can be attained by certain disciplines,
mantras, meditational techniques, and other psychosomatic exercises, without affecting the body in any way, is to put trust in
something that is totally repugnant to our reason.

Considered in this light, any approach to Yoga and transcendental states of consciousness that does not take into account
the biological aspects of the transformation and confines its
attention solely to the miraculous or supernatural elements in
the ancient doctrines can only be classified as puerile. One who
takes such an approach is an obscurantist, indulging in unrealistic fantasies. The wide gulf between some of the modern writings on Tantras and Yoga and the objective realities of this
science has done incalculable harm, not only to the prestige of

this lofty doctrine, but also to the seekers, whose hunger for transcendental experience compels them to devour whatever written material comes their way.

■ *Can you explain what is your idea about Cosmic Consciousness, Superconsciousness, Transcendental Consciousness, and other such terms used to denote higher states of awareness?*

Whenever I refer to any one of these terms, I mean that state of awareness in which consciousness can turn back upon itself and contemplate the Cosmic Reality, apprehended by introspection just as the external world is cognized with the senses and the mind. One of the most distinctive characteristics of this state is that when the individual possessing it turns his attention upon his being, it spreads out and extends in all directions like a drop of oil on a placid sheet of water. There is no limit to this spreading out, and the deeper the contemplation the more extended becomes the area of conscious perception.

When a normal person turns his mind upon himself he finds only the limited periphery of his ego-bound and sense-conditioned awareness. The awakened man perceives his ego and sense impressions reflected in a vast world of consciousness surrounding him on every side. To put it briefly, Cosmic Consciousness signifies an extended state of awareness in which a new area of perception opens within, and consciousness becomes perceptive of itself.

In this connection it is important to bear in mind that in spite of the fact that the quest of the supernatural was pursued even more ardently in earlier times, the law underlying the phenomenon has never been understood. For the ancients, mystical experience or the awakening of *kundalini* represented an entry into divine territory. In their geocentric universe, man appeared as the cream of creation in full development of his capabilities, next in order of precedence to the Creator. Man's concept of a rise in his mental stature could only mean a transition toward a divine order, beyond the pale of human existence, that could release him from the bonds of earth and bring him in close intimacy with the Lord. Today our knowledge of the universe and the realities of life has expanded to such a degree as to show the basic factors underlying such concepts. This idea of gaining access to a higher order of life, free from the fetters of flesh, finds expression in the folklore and myths of almost all the people of the earth. This is also the basis of shamanistic practices and all primitive religious cults. It is therefore easy to understand why seekers of the occult and supernatural undertook arduous disciplines in order to reach a state of blissful incorporeal existence or to win communion with the Lord and Master of Creation.

The fact that miraculous powers have so often been associated with success in Yoga or other forms of religious discipline from remotest times is clear evidence that for the ancients, and even for many people today, these disciplines were and are considered as means of attaining a state of independence, an autonomy free from the ties of the body and mind. They believe that *kundalini* and other forms of Yoga provide an easy way to gain psychic gifts, miraculous powers, or a higher state of consciousness. The connection with body and mind is seldom given serious thought. There is hardly any understanding that for transpersonal manifestations of consciousness the active participation of the brain and the body is essential.

■ *From what you say, Cosmic Consciousness in an individual can be verified by studying certain attributes present in the*

person claiming to have attained to this state. Can there be an
empirical confirmation of these attributes?

Investigation has shown that there occurs a variation in the electrical activity of the brain during sleep and wakefulness. With further development in the methods of science, it may even be possible to distinguish delusive, hallucinatory, and hysterical states by observing variations in the activity of the brain. Perhaps the time is also drawing near when differences in the quality of intelligence and the states of consciousness may also become perceptible. Intensely emotional states in love, hate, anger, happiness, sorrow, and the like are reflected in the body and can even lead to trauma and diseases on the one hand or to buoyancy and health on the other. Extreme suffering and sudden shocks have been known to cause pronounced physiological reactions such as overnight graying of the hair or even sudden death.

Such facts about the body-mind relationship are common knowledge, but they have been overlooked in dealing with mental states associated with Yoga and other spiritual disciplines. Even in the case of those who have not reached a state of mystical union, but in whom the practice of Yoga has been instrumental in bestowing peace of mind, stamina to face the problems of life, a happier inner state or visionary experiences, there must have occurred, however subtle it might be, a physiological alteration in the brain and nervous system to imprint such a change on the personality. If no physiological change has occurred, there is no prospect that the altered experience can continue for any length of time. The expression of mind is so completely dependent on the condition of the brain that it is impossible that any radical change in the former should not affect the latter in some degree. Uncertainty about this vital issue is mainly due to the fact that certain details of the working of the brain and nervous

system, as well as the actual nature of mind, are still unfathomed mysteries.

It is, however, logically consistent to hold that every genuine
form of transcendental experience engendered by any kind of
discipline must be reflected in the human organism and be
attended by subtle or even tangible changes in the brain and
nervous system. If this is conceded, the next step is to study
where the alteration occurs and how it can be detected.

This is an issue of paramount importance for millions who
strive for expanded consciousness. Validation would not only
place mystical experience on an objective basis but also provide
a method for verification and the confirmation of the genuineness of the phenomenon.

From my point of view, therefore, not merely is Cosmic Consciousness a subjective experience, but also it must be attended
by corresponding physiological symptoms. On the subjective
side, the only way to verify its existence is to measure the mental
stature of one who claims it. He must bloom into a spiritual
genius, blessed with *vaikhuri*, the spontaneous flow of higher
wisdom, or *jnana*. On the objective side, he must be an Urdhava-
retas, one in whom the psychic energy has assumed a radiant
form, enveloping his inner being in a never-fading mantle of
light. This is represented in the ancient likenesses of saints and
prophets by a lustrous halo around the head or the body, signifying inner illumination. It is only when the brain is fed by this
radiant psychic energy, changing from white to gold or to the
silvery brightness of the starlit sky, that the otherwise impene-
trable realm of consciousness becomes perceptible to the inner
vision.

A superconscious Yogi cannot continue to have the nervous
system, the brain, or the psychic fuel that nourishes them, of a
normal person. His whole being must be transformed, psycho-

logically and physically, leading to the emergence of a new personality. The subjective and objective verification of Cosmic Consciousness can leave no chance for anyone who is not blessed with this Divine estate to pose as an enlightened being. Because of the prevailing misconceptions, however, it is unfortunately only too common for charlatans desiring fame and power to attract followers who have permitted themselves to believe that transcendental consciousness can be achieved almost overnight by simple techniques rather than by progressive evolution.

In their studies of higher consciousness, the ancient teachers were largely disinterested in the role played by the body, even though the overwhelming effect of some of the physiological changes occurring in the course of Yogic practice left them no alternative but to include them in their writings. They incorporated and correlated them with their own preconceptions about the Divine nature of the occurrences and depicted them in such exaggerated and fantastic colors that, instead of lending corroboration to their statements, they now detract from their value. Even in recent years many individuals credited with expanded consciousness have paid little attention to this important aspect of the occult.

Studied in this light, the ancient Hatha-Yoga manuals will be found to be veritable mines of information about the physiological aspect of the various disciplines. Whether Buddhist or Indian, the Tantric texts also provide valuable hints. The volume of Tantric literature is enormous, and only a fraction of it has been translated into the languages of the West. A good deal of misunderstanding still prevails about this ancient system of metaphysics, and instead of being treated as a handy source for the investigation of mystical experience, these books are often considered to be a storehouse of easy and secret methods of approach to the supernatural. Some treat them even as possible sources of information about methods for the enhancement of sexual potency, prolongation of enjoyment, rejuvenation, and similar ardently desired objectives.

The fact is that out of millions of earnest seekers after Yoga few understand the real nature of the physiological and psychological metamorphosis that has to be effected. The others have their illusions shattered sooner or later after years of hard endeavor. What I claim does not always evoke enthusiasm from those interested in the study of this subject, either for intellectual satisfaction or for self-discovery, because there is still no general recognition of the possibility that the human brain can rise to higher states of consciousness by certain biological readjustments in which the cerebrospinal system plays a decisive part.

2 The Nature of Mystical Experience

■ *What are the essential characteristics of the genuine mystical experience and how can you distinguish it from the experiences caused by mind-altering drugs such as mescalin, hashish, LSD?*

In the first place, mystical experience is overwhelming in a way that transforms the personality. In the majority of cases the experience lasts for only a brief duration. It may occur gradually as the result of Yoga or other spiritual practices or it may come spontaneously to one entirely unprepared for it. In either case the impact is stunning, and the ecstatic feels himself torn from his moorings and face to face with an experience totally foreign to him. It may sometimes take a visionary aspect, involving the form of a Divine Being in glory, or in a Divine order of things. Or one may find oneself transported to other spheres and other-worldly realms.

In the genuine experience the characteristic symptoms are: (1) sensation of light, which can be both internal and external. The subject feels as if a wondrous effulgence has illuminated his interior and maybe even the objects in the outside world. The sensation is at times so realistic as to give the impression of an inner or outer conflagration; (2) an overwhelming sense of wonder and awe; (3) unshakable conviction about the reality of the experience; (4) a sense of infinitude and unbounded knowledge; (5) certainty of immortality; (6) intellectual illumination; (7) a vivid feeling of encounter with an inexpressible, all-knowing Intelligence of an omniscient Divine Being; (8) a flood of pure emotion, an overwhelming feeling of devotion, reverence, submission, love, and adoration, cascading tears, or hair standing on end.

Whether the experience is of a visionary type or unattended by visions and appearances, the most amazing feature lies in the alteration experienced in one's own personality and channels of observation. The observer finds himself transformed. He is no longer the puny, fear-ridden individual, unsure about the nature of his being and destiny. He either realizes himself as a widely stretched, floating mass of consciousness, released from the bondage of flesh, or he finds himself face to face with a celestial being, resplendent and sublime. Or he may see himself surrounded by a superearthly scene of unequalled beauty and grandeur. In almost every case the vision is unlike anything experienced on earth in the ordinary course of life. This feature is so striking that it sharply divides mystical experience from anything seen in dreams or witnessed under drugs.

It is disappointing that there still persists a belief that the altered states of consciousness, brought about by taking drugs like hashish or LSD, correspond in any way to the genuine mystical experience. It should be enough to say that though the latter is inexpressible, one can convey a distant picture by describing it as the highest perfection of grace, beauty, grandeur, harmony, peace, love, rapture, wonder, and happiness, all combined in such an intense degree that the mind may swoon at the stupendous impact of the ecstasy. The drug experience, on the other hand, is exciting and disorienting rather than inspiring. It is not integrated with the normal consciousness and launches the ego into sensational fantasies and distorted perceptions, tending to create addiction and craving rather than creative transformation.

In genuine mystical experience there is often a permanent effect on the mind that has a transforming action on the whole of life. It leads to unshakable belief in the existence of God, even in previously skeptical minds. It also leads to radical change in the pattern of lives formerly devoted to selfish pursuits, resulting in unparalleled acts of altruism, charity, and benevolence, heroism, self-sacrifice, and even martyrdom. It has provided the most powerful incentives for despondent souls for whom the world had ceased to hold any meaning. It has conferred unmatched creative powers on the more advanced recipients of the favor and fashioned them into vessels to enlighten humanity. Research into the religious lore of mankind can corroborate these views.

Throughout the course of history genuine mystical experience has been the mainspring responsible for the progressive growth of human life. It failed to accomplish this only when organized religious institutions barred the way to undiluted mystical experience, forging the chains of dogma and fanatical belief on the adherents of particular sects.

A single test can confirm or falsify my statements. If those interested in the subject would devote their attention to the exploration of mystical experience they will come across a new world of Reality previously unsuspected. If the disciplines of Yoga are given to a hundred volunteers of good intellectual caliber, sound in body and mind, and their reactions observed from day to day for a period of three to five years, unmistakable signs of the awakening of *kundalini* may be noticed in some cases, provided the selection of trainees has been made with due care. The observation of even one case of transformation of consciousness for a reasonable period could lead to remarkable findings and for the first time bring about an understanding of the forces underlying the phenomenon of life.

According to some of the ancient writers who have variously

described it, the transformation leads to the formation of subtle bodies, called *Divya deha* or *Siddha deha*. *Divya deha* means a divine body and *Siddha deha* a perfect one. In every case the reference is to the formation of a lustrous aura round the Self, signifying the radiancy that illuminates the interior of the awakened man. This is by far the most important feature characterizing the consciousness of an accomplished Yogi and the most amazing and fascinating change that he experiences in himself. He now becomes conscious of consciousness itself as a radiant ocean of sentience present everywhere in the cosmos.

After prolonged practice of certain disciplines, some of the candidates may succeed in attaining partial control over their metabolic functions, such as the flow of blood, respiration, or pulse rate. Or they may make themselves immune to pain. But they still may not experience any alteration in consciousness. Some of the Hatha-Yogis in India, who astound audiences with their amazing control over limbs and vital organs, do not possess more than average intelligence and are as remote from enlightenment as any other person. The real test of transcendence lies in the state of consciousness. This fact is of paramount importance and should form the basis of the scientific study and research in this field.

Since a radical transformation in consciousness cannot become possible without transformation of the brain too, it is difficult to predict whether it is possible to detect this alteration with the instruments currently available to science. We know of no mechanical device that can differentiate between the consciousness of a genius and an average individual, although differences in the quality of awareness and insight are obvious. It may not yet be possible to measure the difference in the radiancy or aura of consciousness between an awakened and an average man, either, but with the tremendous progress being made in medical technology, we may be able to do so in the near future.

Apart from the alteration in the brain, there are other physiological characteristics present in varying degrees in mystics and accomplished Yogis that can be detected and studied even with the methods now available. The sphere of activity of *kundalini* is not restricted to enlightened Yogis but also includes men of genius in a positive way, psychic mediums and sensitives in a diluted form, and psychotics in a negative way. The physiological symptoms attending the arousal of the serpent power are present in men and women in all these categories. In making this statement, I fully realize that I enunciate a law that is very difficult for a rational mind to accept without irrefutable evidence, but this proof will, I am sure, be forthcoming at no distant date.

Once it is conceded that human consciousness is capable of exceeding its normal limits and can win to a state of transcendence through the working of certain physiological processes, it follows that these symptoms should also be present, more or less, in the characteristics peculiar to the enlightened state in mediums and highly talented persons. It also follows that since not all attempts at change in nature are successful, there must occur some cases in which the transformative processes do not lead to the desired end but instead result in psychosis and other mental disorders. Thus there are negative as well as positive aspects of *kundalini*. In fact, it is in its universality that the soundness of the hypothesis rests. It would be against the normal course of nature if transcendence or mystical experience were an isolated phenomenon manifested only in the realm of consciousness without other physiological characteristics interwoven with the whole nature of man.

Taking into account the complexity of human nature, the differences in temperament, capacity of the brain, cultural level, religious beliefs, indoctrinated concepts and ideas, it is no wonder that mystical experience shows such a wide variety of forms as observed in the accounts of mystics and seers of all lands. There is unmistakable similarity in basic characteristics of the visionary experience in particular, although the details are so widely divergent.

Because of these differences it is at first difficult to reconcile one account with another and to realize that they all proceed from the same source and the same activity of the brain. This can be observed by comparing the accounts presented by the seers of the Upanishads, the Taoists, Tibetan Yogis, Sufis, Zen masters, and Christian mystics with those who were not under the influence of any particular religious belief but experienced higher consciousness spontaneously without making any special efforts.

The modern seeker after higher consciousness has generally no clear-cut idea about the transcendental condition. Very few have read the original works of the ancient masters, even the Bhagavad-Gita, the Upanishads, the writings of medieval Indian saints like Kabir and Guru Nanak, Sufis like Rumi, and well-known Christian mystics from the past. They usually depend on modern writers and interpreters, few of whom can claim to have had any degree of higher consciousness themselves.

Erroneous conceptions about the ultimate state attained by Yoga are not only prevalent in the West but also exist in the East. There are hundreds of occult sects, creeds, and schools of Yoga and other spiritual systems in vogue today, and the wonder is that the adherents of each believe that their particular system and methods are the best of all, or that their Gurus are among the foremost knowers of spiritual truths. Few disciples ever stop to think that throughout the past the same sentiments motivated and inspired millions of followers of ancient cults that are now obsolete. After a meteoric rise, all fell into decay or were forgotten except for a few isolated followers here and there.

■ *Why is there such a diversity of religious belief and such conflict about the real meaning of religious experience? Is it possible to bring order into this confusion and to achieve unity and harmony among the conflicting faiths?*

There is one major reason why different religions flourish, eventually splitting up into different sects with diverse utterances from their founders, and why there is a recurrent mushroom growth of transient, time-serving cults. In the minds of the people, the supernatural and the divine occupy a place somewhat analogous to that held by fairies, elves, and gnomes in the mind of a child. People believe that by upholding certain doctrines or by practicing certain disciplines they can step from the earth-bound causal existence into a world inhabited by Divine Beings, supernatural entities, and invisible august personages, whose contact can fulfill their hopes and aspirations or inspire and ennoble their lives.

The institutional religions of the world always tried to foster these irrational beliefs. The image of God, the pictures of celestial beings, the delights of paradise, and the terrors of hell were all employed to keep the followers in perpetual hope, suspense, and fear, surrounded by mysterious forces and invisible spirits. The fixation of these ideas through the ages is responsible for the extremely susceptible and gullible state of the mass mind in respect to the Supernatural. It is indeed an anachronism that unrestricted superstition by the mass of people should go hand in hand with the undisguised skepticism of the scholar and the scientist.

The multiplicity of faiths and the recurrent growth and decay of parochial sects and cults can only point to one thing—that the belief in God and the desire to experience higher states of consciousness do not yet stand on a commonly shared solid foundation. The sudden outburst of numerous new cults and novel systems of spiritual discipline on the ashes of the major faiths is but a repetition of a phenomenon that has happened many times in history.

The moment it is established that the religious impulse, or the desire to experience God, is anchored in the organism of man, there must simultaneously occur a change in the existing concepts about the supernatural. Then adherents of one sect or another will no longer be satisfied merely with the assertions of its founders or exponents but will examine and verify their doctrines in the light of the mental and physiological reactions observed in themselves. Similarly, the teachings of Gurus and expositors of the various systems of spiritual discipline will not be evaluated on the basis of their popularity but on the strength of the changes brought about in those who practice them.

If the emergence of a higher state of consciousness is a natural tendency of the mind, then the question that arises is, what is the ultimate object of this impulse and what is the new state of consciousness that it is designed to create? Since the higher state of consciousness can manifest itself only with a corresponding improvement not only in the brain but in the entire organic frame of man, the whole metamorphosis can be so well understood and defined that all those who have had the genuine experience cannot fail to verify it for themselves. At the same time, those who claim to have the experience and come forward to instruct and guide others will not be able to make an impression unless they present their own credentials and establish their claims to the satisfaction of the seekers whom they profess to teach. This would also provide an infallible method of verifying the statements of those who equate the hallucinatory conditions caused by certain drugs with genuine mystical experience. Such experiences are only transitory, abnormal states of consciousness that can be induced and ended at will by altering the chemistry of the nervous system and the brain. Those who make such comparisons reduce religion to a mental aberration, and all the hopes and aspirations of man about immortality and the Divine then become mere figments of his imagination with no basis in reality. In almost all cases, there is no experience ot the beatific state, and they generally base their opinions about it on studies of the experiences of others or on a preconceived image of it in their own minds. Writers like Aldous Huxley and others have been instrumental to a large extent in presenting a distorted picture of mystical experience. Spiritual fiction, like *The Third Eye*, by Lobsung Rampa, a European writer, has tended to create a fantastic picture of the occult and supernatural. Even the most accomplished modern writers on mysticism have not been able to do justice to the experience itself. In spite of their deep interest in the subject, their obvious honesty and purity of purpose, they have not succeeded in conveying an accurate picture of this extraordinary state, for the simple reason that the experience is incommunicable. The inability to present a correct image of their own experiences has been variously expressed by the ancient masters by the use of analogies, as for instance, the impossibility of explaining the nature of light to one blind from birth, or the climax of love to one who has never experienced the ecstasy.

It is no wonder that there is only a distorted or blurred picture of the transcendental experience present in the minds of intellectuals, let alone ordinary people. Among those who write on the subject, very few if any have firsthand knowledge of this marvelous state or even the leisure or inclination to study the self-revelations of the well-known mystics and saints. The false notion that there are distinctive separate forms of the experience for Yoga saints, Zen Buddhists, Christian mystics, Tibetan arhats, and Sufis has further confused the issue and led many

writers on mysticism to confine their attention only to that class
of mystics belonging to their own tradition and faith. No con-
certed attempt has yet been made by a body of dedicated scholars to sift the whole voluminous mass of mystical literature of
all countries in order to find the essential factors common to all
categories. The illogical bias of the nineteenth century against
religious phenomena has been to a large extent responsible for
this chaos in a domain that is virtually the lifeline of humanity.

Genuine mystical experience is rarer than the flash of genius,
and it seems incredible that there should exist so much ignorance about the essential characteristics of the phenomenon.
This lack of precise information, coupled with the exaggerated,
embellished, and even fictitious accounts given by some writers,
makes it extremely difficult to correct the prevailing mass of
misconceptions.

In the genuine mystical experience there is no distortion in
perception, no riot of lights and colors, no unrealistic stimulation of emotions, no unprovoked laughter and no unrelated
sentiments, but an inexpressible transformation of personality.
The precision of the intellect and the accuracy of sensual images
are never lost, distorted, or blurred. On the contrary, the acuity
of perception is heightened, the hues and colors become more
clear and brilliant, the sounds more harmonious, and touch more
sensitive. It is in this state of heightened sensibility and magni-
fied power of perception that the mystic beholds the vision of a
deity, or an external panorama of nature, often completely over-
whelmed by his own highly enlarged power of observation and
the new meaning it gives to every object observed through the
amazing transformation experienced within.

Many of the drugs now in use for effecting alterations in consciousness have been employed for hundreds and even thousands
of years. Certain mushrooms, hashish, peyote, marijuana, and
opium have been in use in South America, India, and China

from time immemorial, and herbal preparations were long used in Africa for hallucinatory purposes. Had there been any identity between mysticism and the drug experience there would at least have been some historical cases of mystics who attained to transcendental states of consciousness through these drugs. Out of gratitude alone, the men so transformed would have themselves acknowledged the source of their inspiration. Of the hundreds of well-known Yoga saints and adepts of India's past, there is not even one in whom the bloom of the mystical state can be traced to drugs. Almost all of them are known to have lived exemplary lives that drew the respect and admiration of the crowds. There is not one work out of hundreds of volumes of inspired writing ascribed to them in which addiction to drugs has been mentioned as a ground for the paranormal stature they achieved. Instead, repeated stress has been laid on the qualities of head and heart that are absolutely necessary to win to the mystical state.

■ *What is the most effective way to induce altered states of consciousness?*

This depends on what is meant by altered states. All states of altered consciousness relate to the condition of the emotions and the mind. The human mind is extremely variable, and it is always prone to change. Strong emotions, such as anger, fear, passion, grief, pain, and anxiety cause changes in our state of consciousness. Illness and disease also cause change. Under the stress of intense emotions men often forget the norms of behavior and at times even act like animals. Most acts of violence and crime are committed in abnormal states of mind. A habitual criminal who delights in robbery and murder may not have possessed a normal state of consciousness from his early life. Our knowledge of consciousness and the action of the brain is so restricted that we often attribute propensity to crime, hysteria, neurosis, paranoia, and the like to some defect in the brain and nervous system or merely to psychic causes.

The real cause, however, is a disproportionate spectrum of *prana*. We know little about *prana*, the ancient Hindu term for psychic or bioenergy, because here we deal with energies and forces beyond the reach of our sensory equipment and the instruments devised to supplement it. Disproportion in the *pranic* spectrum implies disproportion in consciousness. As the result of our evolutionary progress we are now on the threshold of new discoveries in this field. The moment we are able to grasp the nature of psychic energy, we shall be able to deal with abnormal mental conditions and states as effectively as we now deal with abnormal states of the body.

Alterations in consciousness occur also through intoxicants, drugs, excitants, depressants, soporifics, smoking, sleep, fatigue, and the like. Any reagent that can cause an alteration in the *pranic* spectrum can also cause a change in consciousness. The extent and duration of the change depends on the constitution of the individual.

Pharmaceutical research will continue to discover new types of hallucinogens, and the more our knowledge of chemistry grows the more will there be an increase in the number of mind-altering or mind-expanding drugs. The ancients may have known only a few, but there is every likelihood that future drug preparations will be radically different from those in use today. The states of consciousness caused by them may be so exciting and thrilling as to render the existing preparations stale and insipid. Hence those who are attempting to prove that drugs now used can induce states comparable to those experienced in the mystical trance are merely building houses of sand.

It is incredible how shortsighted man can be. The advent of

a more potent and more exciting hallucinogen can cause a revolution not only among the drugtakers but also among those who believe in their efficacy to serve as substitutes for mystical conditions. What they fail to realize is that chemical preparations will continue to change for better or worse, but the mystical experience has been the same for thousands of years and will continue to be the same for ages, until all mankind wins to a higher dimension of consciousness. The altered states of consciousness brought about by drugs, intoxicants, and hallucinogens will always prove to be a chimera, for they will always be subject to change and innovation, thanks to the ingenuity of man and the progress of science.

In order to clarify the point one step further, we should ask how many of those who have studied the effects of these drugs or recommended them to others have experienced the genuine mystical state themselves. If so, what is their description of it? If they never had the experience, how can they honestly assert that the states of consciousness induced by drugs in any way resemble the states experienced in the mystical trance? It is a well-known fact that the alteration in consciousness experienced in mystical ecstasy is so far removed from the normal consciousness as to be inexpressible in the terminology of the latter. The whole religious literature of the world provides unchallengeable testimony to this fact. Almost every great mystic during the last three thousand years who tried to describe his experiences did so only by means of similes, metaphors, riddles, paradoxical descriptions, and even by silence, for here we touch upon realms to which thought and intellect have no access.

It is, therefore, unfortunate that instead of trying first to understand the nature of mystical experience, to define and demarcate it, some writers on the subject, in their haste, should have been instrumental in causing rank confusion in the minds of common people by passing premature opinions and resorting to erroneous comparisons of the genuine ecstasy with the drugged and sodden states of ordinary consciousness.

■ *How then can we distinguish the delusive states of mind from the higher states of consciousness brought about by the awakened kundalini force?*

The answer to this question is not so difficult as might be supposed. In normal human experience, how do we distinguish between sane people and those who are deluded? The same criteria can be applied to the higher state of consciousness. Just as there is a normal pattern for ordinary consciousness so there must be a normal pattern for transcendental consciousness also.

This position is seen in almost all varieties of consciousness exhibited by various species of creatures. Fishes, reptiles, insects, birds, mammals, and human beings all have their own specific patterns of normal consciousness with deeply ingrained reflexes and instincts. If further divided into subspecies and groups, each again corresponds to a particular pattern within the overall frame by which we can distinguish one species from the other. From the lowest animalculae to man, we observe a rigid adherence to this principle of a specific pattern of consciousness for each.

It is only when we come to prevalent ideas about transhuman states of consciousness that there seems to be a radical departure from pattern. Here we find such a variation in the recorded accounts of the world's illuminati that it is difficult to believe that all of them refer to the same experience. In some instances the visionary experiences have been so vivid and realistic that the accounts are most convincing, but they, too, vary from each other.

In the case of most of the Christian mystics and saints, visions of God or the Saviour, angels and devils, heaven and hell, have been common features of their ecstasies. The same holds true for many medieval saints of India, where visions of God or Christ are replaced by Krishna, Rama, or other gods and goddesses of the Hindu pantheon. Among the Taoists, Sufis, and Tibetan saints, visions of the Deity, Buddha, Mohammed, and other divine or superhuman beings, celestial scenes or supernatural occurrences have always been a regular feature of the experience.

These accounts are sometimes in sharp contrast to the descriptions of the transhuman states of consciousness contained in the Upanishads or those rendered by medieval saints of India, such as Guru Nanak, Kabir, Abhinava Gupta, Lalleshwari, Bullah Shah, and others. According to them, the transcendental experience has no resemblance to anything encountered on earth. The same holds true of the Tao of Lao Tse. Many Sufis, like Rumi, describe the state of union of the soul with the universal spirit in the same terms.

In the Bhagavad-Gita the possibility of experiencing the Divine both with and without form has been explicitly asserted. This is also the position taken up in several other Indian scriptures and treatises on Yoga. The view expressed is that God can be experienced by a devotee as attributeless Brahman or as Deity incarnate in the form of Vishnu, Shiva, and so forth. Since the image of God or the Creator is different in different faiths and also varies for the numerous compartments in each faith, the assumption that He can be experienced with form means, in unambivalent terms, that the experience of the Divine with form can be as infinitely varied as there are images and concepts about it in the minds of people.

The classification of the mystical experience into two categories, namely, with form and formless, and the further division of the experience into innumerable categories, corresponding to the extremely varied sects and cults, clearly means the experience has no single specific form or pattern.

It is not only mystical experience with concrete form that provides infinite variations and contrasts, but even the experience of the formless category is not free from ambiguity, for it is not uniform for all saints and mystics of the past. On the basis of the descriptions available, no one can confidently assert that what the Upanishadic seers witnessed in the state is exactly the same as observed by the Buddhist, the Sufi, or the Christian mystics. There is a general similarity, but the experiences do not completely tally with each other.

However, certain characteristics are common to all mystical experience, and we can safely assume that the marked variations with respect to the occurrences and also in the descriptions rendered are through differences in language, traditional religious beliefs, temperament, and mental level of those recording them. In order to be genuine, the basic experience must be attended by the eight unmistakable symptoms described at the beginning of this chapter. If these characteristics are not present in some degree, the experience is delusive. The event itself must be so uplifting and inspiring that it should continue to shine like a beacon through all the vicissitudes and gloom of life. When mystical vision becomes a permanent feature of human consciousness, there is nothing on earth to compare to the glory, beauty, and joy of such a state of being. In contrast, all delusive states constitute a negation of this unimaginable enrichment.

This brings us to a very important point concerning spiritual unfoldment. If spiritual experience actually varied for every faith and cult, then it would represent a singular modification of normal human consciousness peculiar to a certain class—mystics and visionaries alone—and could by no stretch of the imagination be considered to be a universal pattern of higher dimension of consciousness. The reason for this is simple: Since God or the

Author of Creation can have no specific form conditioning Him, and cannot even be formless—for such a state would also impose limitations on His absolute being—it would be irrational to assume that He, Himself, would appear to the devotee in the forms imagined, or in formless aspects. The puny, sense-bound human mind can never comprehend that which is beyond comprehension, the Absolute.

Even though the conditioned consciousness can certainly come nearer to the understanding of the Universal Ocean of Being, of which it is a droplet, this requires the development of a new faculty or channel of perception. The psychophysiological forces responsible for the construction of this channel in us, as a measure of evolution, are those that also create hunger for spiritual experience. It is because this budding channel of higher perception is yet in a rudimentary form, even in acknowledged saints and mystics, that there is so much variation and conflict in the recorded experiences of the ecstatics. Man has still to learn not only how to help in the opening of this Celestial Eye, but also how to maintain that balanced condition of mind and body in which it can function without the least aberration or fault. It is only then that we can formulate a satisfactory description of the normal pattern of higher consciousness and its many variations.

Whatever investigation has been made so far has been directed to accounts contained in the religious literature of the world or available from secondary sources. This has not been a systematic study or a comprehensive one. In the main it has been confined to mysticism as a varied phenomenon, exhibited in various faiths, instead of a critical scrutiny of the avowals of mystics and saints of all periods and places, taken as a whole, with a view to ascertaining the basic factors responsible for the experience. Even a most exhaustive study of this type would not be sufficient to locate the real nature of mystical experience in a way that satisfies the needs of modern knowledge. We have no means of ascertaining that the descriptions on record are not exaggerated or distorted to suit ideas prevalent at the time, or expressing the bias and prejudice of the church or faith to which the authors of the accounts belonged. As the position stands, further examination of these ancient and modern versions of mystical experience cannot now lead to a full understanding of the phenomenon or even to the framing of an overall picture of it that is true for all people and places.

The only way to arrive at a definite conclusion is first to establish beyond doubt the validity of mystical experience. Although the phenomenon has been very rare, we have grounds for believing that certain disciplines and practices, undertaken with a devout frame of mind, can lead to it. We know that such disciplines and practices alone are not enough for success in the enterprise, because even among those who devoted all their lives to the sole aim of gaining transcendence, only a few can be said to have gained their objective. There must be other factors besides the deliberate efforts made by an aspirant that are conducive to success or failure. Though we are not yet in possession of complete knowledge about all these factors, heredity undoubtedly plays a decisive role. Whatever the nature of other unknown factors, certain disciplines and meditational exercises have been instrumental in leading to religious experience in one form or another. How far such experiences were genuine and how far counterfeit we can only estimate by a critical investigation of the accounts available to us.

The only reliable way to discover the nature of the phenomenon is to repeat the methods that led to heightened states of consciousness in the past. This repetition cannot, however, duplicate all the factors involved. For the saint or mystic of the past, arduous preparations, purgations, restraints, and disciplines were necessary to win access to God or Divinity in any form. The aspirant had to cultivate passionate love for the Divine, self-sacrifice, and surrender, and sometimes even resorted to mortification of the flesh under the prevalent idea that the body was the abode of sinful lusts and must, therefore, be treated with severity and held in contempt. Such ideas are still prevalent in some religious quarters. But the modern aspirant who offers himself for the experiment will have a quite different frame of reference and may not be able to cultivate the exact state of mind with which an aspirant embarked upon the quest in ancient times.

For modern experiments it is not necessary to duplicate the environment of monasteries, hermitages, and ashrams. A calm location, free from disturbances and distractions, and reasonably remote from noise and clamor, is all that is necessary for this purpose. The main problem, however, is to procure candidates who have the necessary qualifications that tend toward success. If the number of volunteers is large enough, even the issue of qualifications need not cause obstacles in the conduct of the experiment. There is every likelihood that in a small, healthy group, selected with care, the arousal of *kundalini* may occur in one or two cases. The arousal may not materialize to the extent of causing a complete transformation of personality, or may occur only as a transient phenomenon unattended by significant permanent results. But the metabolic processes generated would suffice to enlighten the investigators to a new potentiality in the human body of which they have not the least suspicion at the present moment. Should a profound transformation occur, they would have before them a repetition of the processes that led to the manifestation of transcendental consciousness in the past. The only differences would be that in one case the processes might have been naturally at work from birth, and in the other stimulated or accelerated by suitable psychosomatic exercises directed to that end. It is not possible that the subjective experience of a successful candidate would completely tally with all the characteristics in the descriptions from the past, but the points of resemblance would be so well marked that there could be no possibility of doubt about the basic identity of the modern experience. This similarity, combined with the psychophysiological changes in the candidate and the readily observable processes set in motion in his system, should satisfy the most critical investigator that the phenomenon witnessed is beyond the present assumptions of modern science.

Considering the radical nature and the far-reaching effect of such transformative processes, even one successful experiment would be sufficient to excite the interest and curiosity of the scientific world. We know that throughout the past almost every case of superconsciousness, whether inborn or attained by religious discipline, has had an almost electrical effect on people who witnessed the phenomenon. Once the possibility of the transformation is established beyond doubt the reaction caused might enormously exceed anything of the sort encountered in the past.

The keen interest evinced now, not only by the common multitudes but also by many scholars in mystical experience, springs from an inherent tendency in the human mind to explore the inner world. One successful experiment would have an effect like that of a match igniting a powder magazine. It may cause a veritable explosion in the thinking of mankind. Once the physiological reactions of an awakened *kundalini* are observed and measured, the repetition of the experiment on an even wider scale would become easily possible. The curiosity excited and the issues involved would be sufficient stimulus for thousands of adventurous spirits to offer their services. It would be necessary for wide publicity to be given to the initial experiment and its results. Like a snowball rolling down the slope of a mountain, gathering mass until it assumes the gigantic proportions of an avalanche, the impact of such experiments on the ranks of skeptics and the rest of mankind are sure to be overwhelming, resulting in the opening of a new healthy channel for the satisfaction of the religious thirst in the searching multitudes.

3   Religion and
Evolution

■ *Do you believe in God?*

I believe in the Eternal Existence, which is the source of our being. God, as conceived in religious systems, particularly in the Semitic faiths, is a personified form of the ultimate or primordial cause behind the cosmos. What I maintain is that it is not possible for man, at his present state of evolution, to apprehend fully the Ultimate, and that even mystical experience or transhuman states of consciousness represent only a brighter state of illumination emitted by the unbounded Sun of Life, which is still at an immeasurable distance from us. The next step on the ladder of evolution may make the illumination even brighter, but the Sun will still be far away. The experience of so-called Cosmic Consciousness, or oneness with the Universe, does not imply a state of identity with the Ultimate but merely entry to a new dimension of consciousness, where the objective world loses its separate existence and assumes the form of a projection of consciousness itself.

Properly speaking, this marvelous experience should herald the utter insignificance of the egobound individuality, on which man prides himself, and an ardent desire to know still more of the amazing world now partially revealed. Instead of treating this as complete union with the Ultimate and hence ascension to a state of sovereignty, one should strive for a higher and still higher experience, for in actual fact there is no limit to the wonders of the beatific state. It is certainly a union with Universal Consciousness, although still restricted because of the limitations of the brain. But the universal Ocean of Consciousness, which is now unfolded before the inner vision of the initiate, is merely the brighter effulgence of an infinite Sun. Heaven alone knows how many steps mankind will rise in the scale of evolution during future millions of years of sojourn on earth, and to what dizzy heights man will continue to soar in the ages to come. To say that mystical experience represents union with God and hence the last milestone in the path of evolution is not only to limit the unbounded glory of the Creator, but also to block the pathway of humanity toward infinitude.

■ *What other reasons do you have for the stand that mystical experience does not represent union with God or the Creator?*

Since the mystical experience depends primarily on a certain enhanced activity of the brain, it is obvious that any state of consciousness, mystical or normal, cannot be the plane of awareness of the Creator, who, even according to current religious concepts, is omniscient, omnipotent, and omnipresent. The human brain is not at all capable of experiencing, even distantly, such an Almighty Being. Further, by the very fact of such a union, any individual who has the experience, to some extent, must partake of these very attributes and himself become omniscient, omnipotent, and omnipresent, at least in relation to the earth, if not to the solar system or the whole of the universe. But, in actual fact, what we see is that even the most enlightened men ever born were not all-knowing, even in respect of their own narrow circle of life, to say nothing of the whole of humanity or the entire organic kingdom on earth. If their knowledge had the least shade of omniscience then they, and not the pioneers of modern science, would have revealed those secrets of nature that have wrought such changes in the life of all mankind.

But in fact they had no inkling of the hidden laws and secrets of matter that were discovered during the last two or three centuries, resulting in the transformation of the earth and the provision of undreamed-of amenities and facilities. It is paradoxical that many of the gifted and talented men who contributed to this amazing progress were either downright skeptics or agnostics. Do we not see the tremendous leap forward taken by Communist countries during the past few decades in the direction of material advancement? Admitting that such progress is one-sided and maybe with side effects of lack of basic freedoms, the fact remains that so far as the world and its problems are concerned, the enlightened mystics of ancient times did not show any greater insight into certain secrets of nature than did those who never claimed communion with God and made no pretensions to oneness with that Omniscient and Omnipotent Being.

■ *But there have been some individuals who claim that because of their own spiritual powers they can arouse the shakti in their disciples and even induce the unitive state in them, so that they too can experience contact with higher states of being.*

Naturally, one who comes in rapport with the Omnipotent Lord must himself acquire some characteristics of omnipotence. I should readily believe that such an individual, by his own sovereign power, would be able to induce higher states of consciousness in his disciples. But in order to provide evidence for the possession of omnipotence, such a person must have power over himself, over his body, over his environment, over the cosmos, and, at least, over his life and death. Have we knowledge of anyone who has attained to such mastery? If so, he or she would be a priceless asset to mankind. If not, how can one assume that one who has not gained mastery over himself or his environment can change the biological functions of another or induce higher states of consciousness in one not mature for the experience?

There are many admirers and followers of spiritual teachers who claim such powers, and about whom it is believed that they are in communion with God or may be an incarnation of God. When the disciples are confronted by events and occurrences that show the extreme fraility and vulnerability of the body of the Guru or Master, they usually defend his alleged superhuman stature by claiming that even the illuminati are subject to Karma, the law of action and reaction in this and future lives. But if their enlightened Guru, in spite of his superhuman stature, is not able to mitigate the effect of his own Karma, how can he do so in the case of others and lead them to expanded states of consciousness?

As is well known, *samadhi,* or the beatific state, implies liberation of the spirit from the bonds of flesh, leading to the cessation of Karma, or bondage and rebirth, according to the manuals of Yoga and scriptural lore of India. The extent to which those in the grip of false beliefs and dogmas can depart from rationality is incredible. How can one ever suppose that a spiritual Guru, who succumbs meekly before his own inflexible Karma, can radically alter or annul the fruit of the accumulated Karma of another and lead him to the ecstatic state, breaking asunder the inexorable causal chain by a mere act of his will, yet remain impotent to do so in his own case?

In order to account for religious experience, we have only a few alternative explanations from which to choose. One explanation can be that the human soul, when filled with an intense desire for emancipation by self-discipline, austerity, penance, worship, meditation, and complete surrender to Will-Divine, evokes a responsive gesture from the Ineffable, which, acting in some mysterious way, leads the aspirant to the beatific vision or, in other words, to a state of union with God. Another is that by all these efforts, including also the special favor of a Guru or the efficacy of a *mantra* or charm, the seeker can take a sudden leap into a miraculous and supernatural world where *vibhutis* (spiritual powers) and *siddhis* (psychic gifts) await his pleasure, and he can employ them for magical and miraculous purposes of his choice. This is more or less the frame of mind of the religious-minded person who believes in the miraculous powers of saints and holy men.

Another explanation is that all mysterious phenomena connected with religion and mysticism are delusory, denoting a hysterical or pathological condition of the brain, or eruption of repressed desires and longings in the unconscious. There certainly are extreme forms of religious belief and practice that clearly savor of hysteria and delusion. To what else can we ascribe the gruesome murders to appease some deity, the mass outbursts of religious frenzy, weird and revolting rituals, sex orgies, witchcraft practices, and satan worship, all reminiscent of once-prevalent, fear-exciting and loathsome savage cults?

Finally, it could be said that there are still unexplored depths in the human brain and that they become active as a measure of evolution, leading to supersensory states of consciousness.

The first alternative can be dismissed on the ground that such a concept is entirely incompatible with the unimaginably sovereign position of the Creator. It is curious how an indefensible idea has kept its hold on the human mind for thousands of years. Why should the Almighty take delight in suffering and make withdrawal from the world, self-mortification, extreme asceticism, or extreme devotion to Himself a precondition for his favor, after having Himself created life with all its frailties and faults, and the world with all its attractions and charms?

Such a combination of egotistic and, we might even say, sadistic traits, would be reprehensible even in an erring creature like man. It is, therefore, the height of folly to associate them with our image of the Almighty Creator. "Cast into the very center of a raging torrent [of passions], bound to a plank [the body], you tell me [O, Allah] to beware and not let even the hem of my robes become wet," says a Persian poet. There can be no stronger refutation of this erroneous point of view than that provided by the amazing advances in science and technology during the past few hundred years, achieved by rational thinking without submission to the dictates of faith.

Had the negation of basic needs or conveniences of flesh, and withdrawals from the world, been natural ideals for mankind to follow under divine ordinance, then we could have never attained the present state of comfort and abundance with the efforts of science. That they have succeeded does not imply a negation of Divinity but only the unsoundness of our narrow views about it.

To suppose that the progress achieved, particularly in Communist countries, signifies the rebellion of man against his Maker, is to ascribe a state of impotency to the Lord, while to hold that such progress is in accordance with the Divine Will and could not be otherwise, at once implies that the emphatic pronouncements and conclusions to the contrary by great pillars of faith have been entirely erroneous and unsound. Do we not now see religious devotees and ascetics, who affect to believe in such erroneous ideas, making full use of the amenities provided by science? They travel in planes and cars, listen to radios and television, wear glasses and hearing aids, use telephones and computers, partake of medicines and modern delicacies, all invented and discovered with great sacrifice and labor by dedicated men who preferred the service of humanity to their own narrow individual salvation.

The second explanation is a direct contravention of what we see in the material and biological kingdoms. It would be fallacious to presume that the human mind is bereft of system, law, and order. In fact, it is the extremely steady and consistent nature of the conscious principle behind the ever-moving mind that enables it to mirror the universe with all its immensity and duration, to weigh and measure it and to mark the working of the immutable laws that rule it. If the conscious mirror were at all uneven, inconstant, or erratic, it would never be possible for the human mind to explore nature and frame a correct picture of it, orderly, complete, and consistent to the minutest degrees. To hold that the world of spirit or universal consciousness is a lawless compound of the magical and miraculous, and that every one who gains entry to it can achieve whatever he likes by merely an act of will, amounts to a negation of all the laws, values, and norms discovered by intellect in the physical world. It would mean a sudden transition into a world of fancies and dreams that has no logic or substance. If union with God betokens a fantastic and capricious dreamworld, then a normal life without such a God-realization is far more preferable and far more salubrious for the soundness and sanity of the human brain.

The third alternative is as delusory and regressive as the phantasmal and delusive states as have been ascribed to religion. It is a sad commentary on the rationalistic trends of this age that pure speculations, without any empirical data to support them, should be allowed to negate a phenomenon that has been a constant feature of civilization from early times and has led to a bloom of talent and genius unparalleled in any other sphere of human thought. Our knowledge of the mysterious forces working in the brain and nervous system of man is too meager to warrant any dogmatic pronouncements about religious experience and the paranormal faculties of the human mind. Those who indulge in intellectual speculation about the nature of mind and consciousness with such a poor knowledge of the brain and nervous system are as guilty of unrealistic flights of fancy as those who have supplied fantastic accounts of the supernatural and the Beyond in the religious literature of the world.

The fourth alternative provides the only plausible explanation for all the varied manifestations of the phenomenon of religion and spiritual experience from prehistoric times to the present day. If a higher divine state of consciousness, partaking to a very limited extent of some of the attributes ascribed by various faiths to Divinity, should be the evolutionary target of the human race, then the appearance of prophets and mystics at different times in various countries, and a hunger for the transcendental, the occult, and the supernatural, deeply rooted in human nature, becomes amenable to a rational explanation without invoking the intervention of a particular god or any other supernatural being.

If the religious impulse and religious experience are the offshoots of an evolutionary impulse, then it is obvious that both must have a biological basis in the human organism that should be empirically demonstrable. In that case, nothing need be taken on trust. The sphere of faith need not then be treated as forbidden ground for the probe of reason. Scientific investigation of the phenomenon ought to be welcomed in order to unfold the secrets of the marvelous transformation that elevated Christ, Buddha, Mohammed, Nanak, and other great prophets to a stature towering over that of emperors and kings. Then the whole literature of mankind, including the various gospels relating to religion, magic, Yoga, and the occult, must be reexamined in the light of this knowledge to discover more about the basic principle underlying them all.

In short, once this explanation is admitted as possessing sufficient plausibility to warrant an investigation, the entire domain of religion and the occult should come under the critical scrutiny of competent observers intent upon resolving the whole phenomenon. When this happens, the present conflict and clash of views about some of the basic problems of life should be automatically resolved, and the true aim of the evolutionary impulse, as also appropriate methods for its acceleration, should be correctly determined.

Considered dispassionately, is it not ironic that instead of acting as a harmonizing factor to unify mankind into one spiritual brotherhood, religion has created an almost irreconcilable fragmentation of humanity? As Jonathan Swift has aptly remarked, "We have enough of religion to hate each other but not enough to love one another." The element of hate and conflict persisted because so many expounders of new faiths claimed finality and infallibility for their own doctrines.

If there is one creator of the universe—it would be ridiculous to suppose that there are several of them—it is inexplicable why there should exist numerous religions, faiths, and cults, each arrogating to itself the position of being the chosen one, each asserting that only its revelation or doctrine is the highest, and each believing that only through the special intercession of its prophet, saint, or Guru, approach to God becomes possible. If the mass of literature of each religion is thoroughly studied, and a comparison is made of the revelations and beliefs expressed by their exponents, it will disclose a state of anarchy in the spiritual realm that has no parallel in any other sphere of human thought. As conditions stand at present, there appears to be no possibility of a complete reconciliation of the various religions of mankind and their fusion into one universal faith, for centuries to come.

■ Where lies the harm if there are many faiths with different

*tenets and different beliefs, each striving for perfection in its
own way to reach God or a higher state of consciousness?
Since there are variations among individuals in their constitutions and mental aptitudes, is it not all the more desirable
to have different faiths to cater to the needs of different
individuals?*

Diversity of creed would not matter if all were agreed upon
the fundamentals, but if there is conflict even about the fundamentals, then it means that the basic issues of religion still lie
unresolved. The question still remains open whether religion at
all has any solid basis or is merely a product of wishful thinking
or of some erratic tendency in the psychological makeup of man.
For instance, some faiths, as for example Buddhism, do not
believe in a Creator. Similarly, there is no agreement about the
concept of God between the various religions. The Brahman of
the Hindus is not really the same as the God of Christians or
Allah of the Muslims. There are also variations about the after-
life and the destiny of individual souls. The law of Karma, which
is a basic tenet of Hinduism, has no place in Islam and Chris-
tianity. How can religious concepts and ideals carry conviction
to the heart when the truth of one is falsified by the other?

Let us look at this issue from another angle. Every religion is
divided into several sects and creeds, and the adherents of each
creed are convinced of the correctness of their own viewpoints.
What conclusion can a dispassionate observer draw from this
fragmentation of each faith into sects and cults? The adherents
are not even agreed among themselves about the tenets and
beliefs of their own faith or, at least, on the interpretations
placed upon them. This, in turn, betokens a state of dissension
that could never arise if the basic issues were beyond question.
The Communist ideology openly repudiates both God and religion, and almost half the world now avows this doctrine. Why

haven't the versatile exponents of religions been able to refute
the Communist dogma to liberate untold millions from the
clutches of disbelief and heresy? Had the world faiths been
united, firm in their beliefs in respect to the fundamental issues,
atheism and agnosticism could never have found room for entry,
much less to enlist the support of half of mankind on their side.

The reason why the current major faiths are not even able to
hold their own against the growing tide of intellectual doubt
and disbelief lies in the fact that the rank and file of each faith
do not stand united in their attitude toward the basic issues of
their own creed. All the faiths, taken together, present such a
sorry picture of rivalry, conflict, and confusion as is utterly in-
commensurate with the alleged sublime nature of religion and
the intellectual stature of modern man. It is only because our
ears have grown accustomed to this pandemonium that we fail
to notice the chaos prevailing everywhere and to realize that if
this state of confusion continues to prevail, the day is not distant
when the whole structure of faith will crumble to dust before
the onslaught of the forces that now stand combined to de-
molish it.

■ *Do you think that investigation into the phenomenon of
kundalini would clear much of the confusion at present prevailing about basic issues of faith?*

One astounding outgrowth of this confusion is seen in the fact
that even in this age of reason, with all the achievements of
technology and advance in education, satan cults and witchcraft
societies should flourish actively even in the most advanced
countries. In India, there have been hundreds of bizarre sects
and cults, ranging from the aghoris, who make no scruple of
eating anything, including even abominable things, to immacu-

late ascetics who are models of virtue and propriety. One can also come across anchorites who live in utter silence and solitude in mountain caves and wildernesses, away from all temptations of the world, in contrast to others who take enormous quantities of drugs, such as hashish and opium, or poisons like arsenic, and still others who indulge in obscene and orgiastic rituals as a religious duty. In fact, since there is no criterion to which one could point with assurance as the hallmark of religious efflorescence, common to all faiths, it leaves the way open for the extremes that have characterized all the religions of today.

Normally when we reflect on religion we usually have before our mind the picture of our own faith and a hazy image of others, but we often fail to visualize the almost limitless variety of religious ideas and concepts, ceremonies and rituals, dogmas and tenets that have held the minds of so many human beings in utter ignorance of the real goal before them. This results in a colossal waste of energy, both mental and physical, of the entire race. If channeled in the right manner, it could lead to as enormous an advance in our knowledge of the occult and the Divine as the advance made in the knowledge of the physical world.

Side by side with saintliness, of which too there are exemplary specimens, there is also such sordidness, squalor, self-indulgence, sadism, self-torture, perversion, disorientation, and depravity associated with religion all over the world as has, probably, no parallel in secular life. Why there should be such horrors side by side with ecstasy and ideals is hard to understand. Some idea of this horror, the antithesis of saintliness and enlightenment, can be gathered from the plight of the impressionable youth who take to promiscuity and drugs in their search for the numinous, ignorant of the fact that the hunger for transcendental experience, unless guided by *viveka* (intellectual discrimination), can lead to the torments of hell instead of to the ecstatic rapture of paradise.

■ Visions of prophets, gurus, superhuman beings, God, Heaven, and Hell and the like have been a constant feature of mystical experience from immemorial times. Aren't they a part and parcel of Superconsciousness?

It is perfectly correct to hold that visions, extremely varied in nature, have been an almost inseparable feature of mystical consciousness. Among the primitive shamans, visionary experience was common. In fact, apparitions of superhuman beings and unearthly creatures formed the basis of their religious experiences. Believing, as many people do even today, that mystical experience denotes direct communion with God or other heavenly beings, visions and apparitions automatically seem a natural outcome of their religious experiences. What stronger proof of Divine favor could a devotee expect or long for than the actual realization of his self-formed image of God, or other superhuman beings, during the course of his meditation or worship? It is no wonder that those who achieved such visions as the culminating reward of years of extreme self-denial and austerity were so transported that they forgot the world and its allurements in the rapt contemplation of the adored beings.

This is certainly not surprising, considering the fact that in the heightened state of consciousness engendered by an awakened *kundalini*, visionary experiences become much more pronounced. The whole iconographic system of Hatha-Yoga is based on this possibility. The sadhaka, or aspirant, at the commencement of his practice, learns to visualize the upgoing current of *kundalini*, the *cakras* with their lotuses and letters of the alphabet, their presiding deities, sounds of *mantras*, the hues and colors connected with them and other imaginary objects relating to the system. When the awakening actually occurs and consciousness is expanded, the visions become even more vivid and realistic. A similar condition occurs with the action of hallucinogenic drugs and hypnosis. We can therefore reasonably expect proneness to visionary states in one with an awakened *kundalini*. An extreme form of this hallucinatory tendency is also found in psychotics, a product of *kundalini* active in a morbid way. Vivid and heightened imagery, whether visual or auditory, is also often a marked feature of a genius.

It is, therefore, but natural that one in whom *kundalini* has generated a highly expanded state of consciousness should be prone to visions of some sort where the pattern is already set by the ideas and notions habitual to him. But it is important to remember that all these visionary experiences with shape, form, place, or time are but the figments of one's own imagination, rendered vivid and realistic by the radiant stream of *kundalini*. The gods and goddesses, angels and devils, heavens and hells, superhuman and subhuman beings, strange unearthly creatures, astral and mental planes, conditioned by earthly time, space, name, form, or figure, have no real significance, but are merely the creations of the subjects themselves through their active and glowing imagination.

The higher state of consciousness, despite its enrapturing radiancy and the alluring sounds in the ears, is as void of visions and hallucinatory figments as the consciousness of a healthy, wise, and clear-thinking human being, who calls a spade a spade, and who views everything he comes across in sane perspective and proportion, always ready to distinguish reality from a dream or a hallucination.

■ *Does this mean that visions and hallucinations are necessary accompaniments to higher states of consciousness and that the future man will be more liable to phantasmic states of mind than we are?*

Normal human beings or, for that matter, any other forms of life, from the lowest to the highest, are not generally prone to visual fallacies and hallucinations. How then can false appearances be an ornament of a superconscious mind? Among average people, liability to visions and hallucinations is extremely rare, its greatest incidence being among hysterics, neurotics, and the insane. Another category that is more liable to hallucinations is that of drug addicts. A normal, healthy human brain allows no room to hallucinations, spectral appearances, or ghostly apparitions, for the very sound reason that such a state of mind would seriously interfere with its capacity for survival. It is hardly likely that one prone to visions and hallucinations can be master of his own actions and thoughts. On the contrary, the person subject to them is likely to be a slave to his fancies and to the fantastic appearances created by his mind. The same holds true for all other forms of life. Even a slight aberration of mental faculties, if permanent, can be more lethal to survival than a serious disorder of the body. The mentally disordered become wholly incapacitated for the battle of life and are seldom trusted with responsible duties. One with an unbalanced mind does not command confidence, even among his friends and family. He has their sympathy but not their trust.

Those who lay claims to visionary experiences or encounters with superhuman beings and unearthly creatures, and treat them as a commendable feature of transcendence are, perhaps, never cognizant of the fact that save for people of hysteric, neurotic, and psychotic categories, the great bulk of the race is completely free of phantasmic states of mind. This being so, it means that such visionaries, by their own admissions and confessions, of which they are often highly proud, create a gulf between themselves and the sane majority of mankind. Since the existence of an anthropomorphic God as the creator of the universe, who appears to His devotees in personified forms in visions, is logically out of the question, in view of the colossal dimensions of the cosmos, one cannot doubt that such visions and appearances in the mystical state are conjured up by the visionary's own highly susceptible and powerful imagination and have no actual basis in reality. They serve the useful purpose of wish fulfillment much in the same way as dreams sometimes do in the case of normal human beings.

In certain exalted cases, such visions are a kind of emotional poetry of the soul, similies and metaphors of the illimitable and incommunicable, which are not to be taken literally.

I am making these statements with a full sense of responsibility, knowing that visions and voices from the void form a considerable portion of the narratives of mystical experiences recorded by saints and seers of all periods and countries. Visions play a great part, especially in the case of Christian mystics and the Vaishnavite devotees of India. Most of the great mystics of the world tell us in devout and convincing terms of their rapturous communion with the adored Savior, God, Goddess, or other Divine Beings, the transports of joy that they felt and the communications they received from them. Modern writers on mysticism have accepted these stories as a valid phenomenon of the beatific state or as a possibility arising out of the fact that Divinity, although purely spiritual in nature, without name and form and hence inapprehensible, must assume some form or shape in order to materialize before the inner eyes of the devotee as a gesture of grace to bring conviction to an ardently seeking mind. For them, therefore, visionary experiences are a necessary corollary to the struggle of an aspirant for God-realization.

It is true that from the point of view of the major faiths of mankind, spiritual experience is regarded as a mark of Divine favor or a culminating point of sustained efforts for emancipation carried on for years or even for several lives. The occurrence of visions and hallucinatory trance states appears as a natural consummation of the practices and disciplines undertaken. But there are other faiths and systems of metaphysics, according to which mystical experience does not necessarily imply a spiritual intercourse with God or a Divine Creator of the universe.

For instance, according to the Sankhya system of Hindu philosophy, the human soul, by righteous modes of conduct and religious practices, gains freedom from the enfettering bonds of prakriti or matter and realizes its own glorious, immortal nature. According to Mahavira, the founder of Jainism in India, spiritual experience denotes liberation of the embodied soul from the chains of flesh and brings visions of the soul's own glory and the glory of other exalted souls known as Tirthankars. For Buddha, cessation of the cycle of births and deaths, and entry into an inexpressible, painless state of Nirvana, represents the consummation of a well-spent, righteous life.

Even the Brahman or Absolute of the Upanishads is not Godhead in the sense used in the Semitic faiths. It is the Reality behind the phenomenal world, the conscious substratum of all the endlessly variegated creation apprehended by our senses and the mind. The human soul, divested of the limitations imposed upon it by *maya* or illusion, is verily Brahman itself, entire and whole, without any attribute of form, size, smell, touch, sound, and taste, an unimaginable and indescribable Reality, designated emblematically by the term "Sat-Chit-Ananda," Existence, Consciousness, Bliss.

The same applies practically to the attributeless Shiva of the Shaivites. For them, the embodied Jiva or individual soul is a drop from the ocean, which is Shiva himself. For the Vedantins, it is a spark of the fire which is Brahman. Several of the Christian mystics, as for instance, Master Eckhart, Dionysius, St. Marcus of Egypt, and St. John of the Cross, clearly express their identity with Godhead. Several of the eminent Sufis, like Rumi

Baba Kuhi, Attar, Al-Hallaj, and others, express themselves in the same way.

With mild variations in cosmogony and methods of approach, most of the well-known medieval saints and mystics of India upheld the view about the identity of the embodied human soul and the creative consciousness. Where the identity is not clearly acknowledged, the relationship of father and son, master and servant, or mother and child is substituted. In every case, the existence of an unbreakable bond of kinship between the Almighty and the human soul is always acknowledged. The same idea is expressed by Christ when He says that He and his Father are one.

This leads us to a crucial phase in our consideration of the norms of mystical experience. Whatever view is taken—whether the human soul is considered to be identical with the attributeless Brahman, Shiva, Allah, God, or Jehovah, or whether it is treated as a self-existing pool of consciousness as in Sankhya, Jainism, or Buddhism, in a Godless world, or as the son, servant, or creation of God—the one important fact that emerges from all these varied definitions and religious doctrines is that the soul can only be spiritual in nature without form, size, shape, and name. Therefore, in this respect it partakes, to a lesser extent, of the nature of the attributeless Universal Spirit or the Absolute. Whether we take a monotheistic, dualistic, or pantheistic view of creation, or whether we treat the human soul and the Cosmic Reality as identical or separate, in the form of the Creator and the created, the spiritual nature of the Maker or of the human soul can in no case be denied. Belief in any one of the major faiths, or even in any one of their sects, simultaneously involves belief in the spiritual nature of the human soul. Even where the existence of God or the Creator is denied, belief in the immortality and spiritual nature of the soul is readily admitted.

Belief in the spiritual nature of the soul means belief in its incorporeal existence without any of the appendages imposed on it by embodiment. Even the primitive believed in the immaterial nature of the discarnate soul. The area of conflict, however, begins to appear when we try to translate this idea into human terms. The point is, can we frame a picture of the soul or, in other words, of the human pool of consciousness in the discarnate form? We can certainly dimly picture an "area of awareness" like our own and suppose that this should be the intrinsic disembodied image of the soul, but how can we supply any form to it or locate it in time or place, when in the discarnate state it is totally cut off from every sensory perception? Can we even supply a form to our own consciousness?

Again, according to the tenets of existing faiths, every human being has in him the possibility, with a rightly spent life and certain disciplines, of gaining approach to his Maker, to the Cosmic plane of Consciousness, or to the hidden depths of his own soul. This points to a universal belief, expressed in all great religions, that man can ascend to a higher plane of consciousness either in his rapturous contact with God, Brahman, or Allah, or in the unfoldment of his own hidden possibilities and realization of his own deathless and glorious nature.

Although there are conflicts and variations about this concept, and even about the existence of the Creator, there is a general agreement among the various faiths about the sublime destiny of the soul. What other idea can this universal belief convey to us except that all great founders of religions and all true sages instinctively had a feeling that man was destined for a brighter and more glorious state of being than his present existence? The only point of difference lies in that this glorious state was visualized as being solely due to the union with God or Universal Consciousness, and not also to the physical cause, a biological transformation of the brain and nervous system leading to the emergence of a blissful and expanded state of consciousness, the natural endowment of future man. There was little appreciation that what all the systems of religious discipline promise is actually being slowly developed in every human being as the result of irresistible evolutionary processes.

The visionary aspect of mystical experience cannot be a lasting feature of the future expanded consciousness of the race for two reasons. Firstly, because such a state of consciousness would pose a threat to its own survival in a strictly causal world, and secondly, because susceptibility to visions and apparitions would never allow that uniformity in observation, clarity of expression, and homogeneity of ideas that enables the human intellect to draw precise conclusions from observed data. A loose state of consciousness, subject to divine and spectral visionary experiences, if a common feature of the mind, would only result in the establishment of a capering and gesticulating bedlam on earth. The visionary aspect of superconsciousness can, therefore, be only a transitory feature, attendant on a process of development in much the same way as myth and superstition constituted a prominent symptom of the primitive mind during the course of its ascent toward a fuller flowering of the intellect.

My only major point of departure from the accepted religious traditions of all lands lies in that I ascribe the emergence of higher states of consciousness—whether caused by any form of religious discipline or occurring spontaneously—to an *evolutionary metamorphosis* slowly taking place in the race through cosmic laws of which we have no precise understanding at present. This slow progression toward a wider state of consciousness is as predestined as was the rise of man from animal to human consciousness. And it is as much in accordance with the will of the Creator as primary evolution. One great difference between the two is that man, a self-conscious being, can by his own efforts and contribution accelerate or retard the processes now at work to invest him with the already mapped expanded state of consciousness. This is the only rational explanation that can be placed upon the extraordinary events of history caused by those exceptionally gifted men and women who claimed communion with God or higher planes of consciousness as the authority for their thoughts and actions throughout the past.

When once we concede that the founders of religions and other well-known seers and sages were peculiarly constituted men and women prone to spiritual experience, this also involves the admission that their brains and nervous systems must have been more attuned to subtle vibrations of intelligent energies to which an average brain is unresponsive. We will also have to admit that this peculiar constitution of the brain and nervous system cannot be basically different in different individuals, for the reason that all natural biological functions and rhythms tend to be uniform in the same species or groups. This means that if there is a definite evolutionary impulse at work in the race, the processes leading to it and the goal in view must be uniform for all human beings.

We can therefore assume that the visions and hallucinations —whether visual or auditory, or of any other sensory nature, that are extremely divergent, varying from individual to individual— must be the creations of the individual mind and not the natural result of the evolutionary processes. Otherwise they would be necessarily uniform and undifferentiated in character. The opinion sometimes expressed by those investigating the effects of hallucinogenic drugs that they resemble the visionary experiences undergone in mystical states clearly rests, therefore, on an error. Mystical experience must either be the product of a peculiarly constructed brain or the result of altered chemistry of the body, or a hallucination. There is no other alternative to explain all the facts. If the experience is real, it must have roots in the organic constitution of the brain. If the brain is of the normal pattern and the experience is due to a sudden biochemical alteration, as in the case of drugs, then the whole experience is superficial and transitory and has no basis in reality.

What, then, is the significance of the visions and ecstasies of mystics? When we admit that a regular biological process is at work in the brain to invest it with an expanded state of consciousness, and that in the case of mystics and saints this process is either more active from birth or highly accelerated by means of intense psychosomatic exercise, then it is easy to see that the emergence of the higher state of consciousness with complete clarity and precision cannot be possible all at once. Like other processes of growth, it must be attended by ups and downs, diversions and distortions, to be smoothed out and straightened in the course of time. Visions and hallucinations occur in the intermediate stage before the brain is completely attuned to its higher functions. We come across the same diversions and distortions in the growth of the human mind from infancy to adulthood. Since the child is not self-conscious or only dimly conscious of itself, it accepts these fluctuations in its mental development as a matter of course without understanding or even noticing them.

In the case of an adult who suddenly finds himself confronted by another dimension of consciousness, the understanding has to occur in one form or other to save him from perplexity and confusion. In view of the obscurity and secrecy that veils the supernatural and the divine, it is well-nigh impossible for a human being, brought face to face with the inexplicable and overwhelming transcendental experience, to apprehend immediately that he has entered another dimension of consciousness and that a wondrous new world has been opened before his inner vision. If his higher self—now unfolding itself before him in all its glory, filling him with happiness, awe, and wonder—does not project itself in conformity to his preexisting ideas and concepts in a visionary experience of some sort, the chances are that he would be completely lost, bewildered, and confused. To some degree this actually happens in the case of those in whom the sudden awakening of *kundalini* is attended by mental derangement of some kind.

■ *What you state implies a departure from the views expressed by the greatest spiritual teachers of humanity, most of whom were inspired. Do you mean to say that their knowledge was imperfect and the biological basis of the experience escaped their attention?*

I have the greatest reverence for all the great spiritual teachers of the past. Had any one of them, for instance, Vajnavalkya, Buddha, Socrates, Vyasa, Christ, Shankara, or Plotinus, been born in the present age of expanded knowledge, he would have immeasurably excelled me in presenting spiritual truths in the light of what mankind has discovered since then in the sphere of biology and other sciences. I would not even be able to hold a candle to him. Judging from the level of knowledge prevalent in their day, every one of these great teachers was a prodigy of the highest order. The tragedy has been that the knowledge of the physical world and in particular of the human body was extremely limited in their day and the whole atmosphere vitiated with wrong ideas, myths, and superstition. Moreover, their followers and interpreters, treating their utterances as the final word on the religious aspirations of man, formed their teachings into a stationary pool instead of a flowing stream, gathering rivulets of fresh water to renew it and save it from stagnation until it could become a river to quench the thirst of all humanity.

I am but the mouthpiece of relentless time. The ideas I am expressing are inevitable at this point of human progress. There is every chance that some investigators, working independently on consciousness or on the causes responsible for psychoses or even psychic phenomena, will ultimately come to the same conclusions that I have drawn. I do not in the least arrogate to myself a position superior to that of any of the great spiritual luminaries of the past. On the contrary, I regard them as my masters and initiators on the path. Without the treasures of thought bequeathed by them, I could never understand my own extraordinary experience nor have had the courage to express my views with confidence, for I would utterly lack the confirmation of my own experience that their works provide. We have only to visualize the dark clouds of superstition and ignorance overhanging the minds of people of their time to realize their colossal stature and the brilliant light they shed for the guidance of mankind.

Human knowledge, like a child, has to grow resistlessly to a predetermined stature in keeping with the evolutionary progress of the race. No efforts by religious zealots or fanatics in any branch of knowledge to impede its progress or to divert it into parochial channels can meet success for long. Like a turbulent flood sweeping away the embankments erected to restrain it, fresh waves of thought, issuing from brains adjusted to the evolutionary need of the race, will wash away the walls erected by dogma and fanaticism in the spheres of both religion and science.

I am but expressing the truths taught to me by my own experience, originating from the same source from which the seers and sages of the past drew their inspiration. What I assert is in answer to the call of time. After proper experiments are made and the truth of what I say is empirically established, it will be possible to understand the needs and demands of the time that made this disclosure of a mighty law of nature unavoidable at this juncture. Every human being draws his life, his breath, and his wisdom from the same Infinite Source of knowledge, and

Destiny decrees the part that every one of us has to perform. Somehow the disclosure of this still little understood law of nature fell to my lot.

It is for this reason that I am so emphatic about the imperative need of an investigation into the phenomenon of *kundalini*. There can be no greater error than to suppose that the present distorted and erratic trends in religion, and the subversive and regressive currents in social and moral ideas that have now spread over the world, will disappear or automatically correct themselves with the passage of time. Those who view this anarchy and the erosion of accepted values with grave concern should prepare themselves for a further progressive deterioration of the situation, unless it is empirically established that ethical upliftment is an inseparable part of human evolution. It is not man's own choice or the exigencies of his social life that make morality desirable; but a virtuous life is an essential part of enlightenment, an indispensable ingredient of evolutionary growth.

The discontentment and the revolt of modern youth does not spring merely from an intellectual dissatisfaction with existing values and norms in the spiritual, social, or political fields, but also from a subconscious recognition of a vicious environment, inimical to the evolutionary progress of the race. No amount of haranguing from the pulpit or persuasion in the press, no amount of exhortation in scholarly works, and no amount of legislation will help to arrest the growth of this canker unless the evolutionary demands are fulfilled and the errors rectified.

Investigation into the phenomenon of *kundalini* will bring to light three cardinal issues about which the world at large is at present completely in the dark. The first to come under scrutiny will be the discovery that the reproductive system also acts as the evolutionary mechanism, and that the human brain already has in it a potentiality to express a higher dimension of consciousness when fed by a more potent form of bioenergy for which the system is already prepared. The second is that the religious impulse is based on inherent evolutionary tendencies in the psyche, and that the reproductive-cum-evolutionary mechanism exerts a pressure on the brain, creating an urge for religious experience in a way similar to that which causes the expression of the sexual impulse at puberty or earlier in all normal men and women. The third issue of paramount importance will be that it would make clear beyond the least doubt that there is a predetermined target for the evolution of man, and the whole race is being irresistibly drawn toward it.

I have no words to emphasize the importance of this demonstration. All our current ideas and notions about progress, all our present systems of philosophy, all our views about ideal social and political orders, all our concepts about religion and the Beyond, and all our opinions about ethics, about right and wrong or good and bad, will shrink to a subordinate position before this Revelation. If the whole organism of man is evolving inexorably toward a certain predetermined target, it means that there is no other problem so pressing and no other need so urgent as to determine the direction and the ultimate goal of this evolutionary drive in order to live in harmony with the inherent dynamics of our being.

When it is conclusively demonstrated that all religious ideas and concepts, all rituals and ceremonies, and all modes of worship and prayer owe their existence to an inherent evolutionary impulse at work in the human body that cannot be thwarted or obstructed with impunity, it should bring mankind toward a frame of mind in which the observance of the laws and the principles governing the activity that can lead to the realization of spiritual ideals will become as inseparable a part of our daily life as the observance of the laws and principles of hygiene at present.

We can easily recall the time when a similar conflict of views and confusion prevailed about the cause and nature of diseases invading human flesh and the methods to combat them. This provided a great opportunity for charlatanism and quackery. There was no end to fantastic views about the causes and treatment of contagious diseases, each healer handling his patients in accordance with his own favorite and sometimes even bizarre theories. Belief in the efficacy of foolish and even obnoxious remedies, such as the raw flesh, blood, and even excreta and urine of certain unclean animals and birds, strangely compounded potions and philters, and faith in amulets, magical devices, and the like, were rife everywhere. But when once the basic facts concerning certain common diseases like pneumonia, malaria, typhoid, tuberculosis, and so forth, were known and methods to fight infection and contagion devised, the whole system of therapy underwent a change. Although there are still many gaps and problems, there is a workable unanimity about the basic principles, and this has led to the systematization of the theories and the methods of treatment of various diseases. The result is that the confusion and chaos that once prevailed in this most important branch of human knowledge has to a large extent ceased to exist.

■ *There are at the moment hundreds of spiritual cults and creeds, and hundreds of different systems of spiritual discipline and mind culture, each bearing the hallmark of one spiritual teacher or the other. Does the existence of these numerous cults and creeds and diverse systems of discipline help mankind in the transition you envisage, or do they constitute an obstacle in the path?*

I think that they are still a definite help in the process of transformation I am describing. The summary dismissal of religion as a subject not worthy of attention on the part of some over-critical luminaries of the last two centuries—oblivious to the importance of spiritual ideals and beliefs—has created a vicious climate of skepticism and disbelief that is highly dangerous for the survival of the race. No degree of luxury and no store of material allurements can keep the evolving mind of men tied forever to earth. Sooner or later it must break its tether to soar to the golden heights of self-knowledge for which it is destined. The revolt against the existing order—the indiscipline rampant everywhere and the sudden distaste of youth for the standards and values of their parents and grandparents—is the outcome of the all-out efforts of the evolving mind to break the chains forged by a narrow-minded philosophy of life followed by some of the architects of modern society. They believed that mankind could manage very well all by itself without having its mind fettered by the supernatural and the divine.

Every existing religion, faith, or spiritual discipline acts, to a greater or lesser extent, as a bulwark against the advancing tide of rank materialism unleashed by skeptical intellect. It is a tragedy that the fathers of modern materialistic thought could not foresee the disastrous consequences of their hasty conclusions, and it is even more tragic that such conclusions, backed by a ponderous show of learning, should have been so readily accepted by others, even against their own better judgment or intuition. Even now there is little realistic cognizance that no power on earth can prevent the mind of man from being occupied with orgies of violence and crime when once it is deflected from the evolutionary target toward which it is bound. Therefore any effort made to throw cold water on the spiritual aspirations of the masses—to imprint on their minds the false idea that there is no spiritual order in the universe and no sublime goal toward which they have to strive—is to change the direction of their thinking from sublime to lowly objectives, diminishing their enthusiasm for a noble life.

Some inveterate skeptics, confronted with this accusation, will no doubt point to statistics to show that from an ethical point of view, people in the past, when they were firmly in the grip of religious belief, were no better than they are now. But in advancing this argument they often forget that if we had lavished even a fraction of the attention devoted to the transformation of the physical environment to the spiritual side also, the improvement in the mental atmosphere effected would have made the world a far more peaceful, far more secure, and a far more joyful place to live. The still surviving faiths provide at least some sort of spiritual food for the hungry crowds, serving to keep the mind holding on to its evolutionary target, however imperfectly depicted it may be, and to save it from being cast into a yawning gulf of anarchy, totally cut off from the saving light that keeps it healthy and sane.

■ *But don't Russia and China provide outstanding examples of the success of a materialistic ideology?*

The period of trial of the methods adopted in both the countries has been too short to draw definite conclusions. But already we have clear indications before us to frame a picture of the unsafe position the world would assume if all the nations of the world followed the same ideologies. It is hardly necessary to stress the ruthless repression, purges, and bloody massacres that occurred in Russia and other Communist countries, because there have been similar gruesome episodes in other lands as well. But one thing is evident, that the main objective of the founders of communism, to build a classless, happy, and strife-free society, has not been achieved. Already China is accusing Russia of revisionism and imperialistic tendencies. In another one or two decades China itself may become the target of similar criticism from sister countries professing the same ideology. The one important lesson that the experience of the last few decades imparts is that, whatever the political order and however rich a country might become because of it, there occurs no diminution in the fires of lust, passion, hate, and envy smoldering in the human heart, and that they can leap into destructive flames at the slightest provocation whenever an opportunity presents itself.

The human mind can never abide in a state of contentment and peace, even if the wealth of the earth and all the amenities that human ingenuity can devise are placed at the disposal of each individual, unless the evolutionary target is attained. When it has everything it needs for a luxurious life, then, unless there are noble and sublime aims before it, it will hanker after power, sovereignty, sex, name and fame, and other ambitious objectives. Nor do nations that grow to wealth and power abide contentedly with what they have achieved; they never cease to strive for ascendency and domination over other nations. After gaining ascendency on earth, if possible, they would strive for conquest of other planets wherever they found possibilities of habitation to serve as an object of their territorial ambitions. The Communist experiment achieved a certain measure of success because of its basic tenets of economic and social parity. Equality of opportunity for all human beings, abolition of want, and removal of dependence are also some of the fundamental needs of evolution. It will fail because it provides no sublime ideal for man's restless mind, and indeed actively prohibits freedom of thought. The religions of the capitalist societies fulfill the need for ideals to some extent, but they are often overshadowed by materialistic greed and do not often act upon the basic tenets of the creeds that they profess. They need revision to come into harmony with the needs of the evolutionary impulse and the present intellectual stature of mankind.

Many kingdoms and empires of the past achieved a great

measure of success and dominated the world for centuries, only to fall victims to degeneration and decay. Phenomenal success in the initial stages of a new doctrine or ideology is no guarantee of its lasting worth, but, on the contrary, may even be a symptom of early decay. No political or social system that is not in harmony with the evolutionary needs can survive the onslaught of time. The doctrines of the major faiths of mankind survived for many centuries because the ethical and spiritual teachings they inculcated were more or less concordant with the demands of the evolutionary force. All these faiths have now lost their dominating position because the Communist ideology made use of their basic principles—while those who ostensibly follow religious faiths often in practice spurned these noble ideals, attaching far greater importance to the outer formalities, to the husk rather than to the kernel of their creeds.

The human race cannot afford any longer to experiment with this or that political ideology. The whole earth has now been transformed into one vast arsenal that, through the slightest error of an imprudent political head—or the deliberate intent of another with a sadistic bent of mind, or the caprice of a third—can explode instantaneously, spelling the doom of the entire human race. The only way to safety and survival lies in determining the evolutionary needs and in erecting our social and political systems in conformity with those needs. It is not wise to use the word "success" for any political ideology at a time when mankind is virtually trembling on the brink of the greatest catastrophe of all time.

■ *Will the race face any danger in the near future if the laws of kundalini are not understood and determined?*

Certainly neglect or violation of any laws of nature is always fraught with danger. This is especially true of the still obscure laws of life. Our present picture of the universe has to be extended to include intelligent energies and forces surrounding us and sustaining the processes of life to which we owe our existence and all our spheres of activity, although they are not cognizable through the senses. Every breath that we draw, every involuntary impulse or activity of our body, and every metabolic and catabolic process, working within us, is not caused by the atoms and molecules in our flesh, but by subtle, intelligent forces that work unseen all around. Every human being, every animal, and every plant is the handiwork of an all-pervading, tireless, intelligent energy that is the architect of all embodied life in the cosmos. The universe that we see is a vast storehouse of amazing superphysical energies and forces, besides the material energy perceptible to our senses, but we are insensitive to them, as one who is color-blind is unappreciative of the infinite variety of colors surrounding him in a blooming flower garden.

The aim of the evolutionary impulse that is active in the race is to mold the human brain and nervous system to a state of perception where the invisible world of intelligent cosmic forces can become cognizable to every human being. Can there be any more powerful factor to remind us that we are in a state of constant transition toward an unknown destination than the picture of our primitive ancestors of less than ten thousand years ago, working with instruments of flint to fashion their weapons and implements of stone, living in caves, sheds, or skin tents in a rough, savage way of life so abhorrent to our present tastes that, even if experienced in a dream, may cause the horrors of a nightmare? With the transition that has occurred clearly before our eyes, we can easily infer that not even in their wildest fancy could those leading that barbaric mode of life imagine their distant progeny in the present state of glamor, abundance, and luxury we enjoy today. With this example clearly before our mind, can there be a greater instance of purblindness than ours if we, in turn, fail to realize that in the next, maybe one or two thousand years, our descendants may present a vastly different picture, almost as different as we present now in comparison to our ancestors of the neolithic age?

The evolutionary mechanism, carrying us toward this unknown destination, with full awareness of the target to be achieved and full knowledge of all the infinitely complex biological changes necessary to attain this end, must be, as we can readily imagine, guided by a Superintelligence, beyond anything that we can conceive in human terms. In fact, any cosmic scheme of planned evolution presupposes the operation of an Intelligence aware of every detail of the universe past, present, and future. In the conditioned sphere of embodied life, the resistance offered in thought or deed by self-conscious human beings to the inner processes working toward that predetermined end cannot but react adversely and even violently on those guilty of transgressions. The importance of Revelation has lain in this, that it is the only channel open to mankind to know step by step the modes of behavior and the ways of thought necessary in order to live in consonance with the still hidden evolutionary laws. Except for this one single important objective, Revelation can have no other meaning or significance whatsoever, and could never win the adherence and homage that it commanded for thousands of years in all faiths. This is the only rational explanation to account for the tremendous influence exercised by the revealed scriptures of the world and the mentally dominating position occupied by the various faiths that made use of the teachings inculcated for the guidance of their followers. At the present moment, we are passing through one of those crucial periods in human history when collective breach of the evolutionary canons has attained to such a proportion that catastrophes appear imminent unless the transgression ceases before the saturation point.

4 Yoga and Higher Consciousness

■ *Can you say why there is a general impression prevailing that there are hidden methods by which success in Yoga or other occult disciplines becomes easy to obtain?*

If the state of mind desired to be achieved by the practice of Yoga is a higher state of consciousness, based on a biological reconstruction of the brain, it is idle to expect that there can be any secret methods that can instantaneously cause this transformation. There are cases where people attained to ecstatic experiences suddenly or after only a short practice, but the quickness of results in such cases was more due to a ripe condition of the brain and nervous system for the experience than to the efficacy of the methods employed.

It is to be borne in mind that *kundalini* as the evolutionary impulse in the race is perennially active, but this activity is so slow and based on so many factors, that it is almost imperceptible and is constantly in a state of flux. It is only when, through the normal activity of the evolutionary mechanism, the brain and nervous system have reached a certain state of maturity that only a slight or moderate effort is needed to lead to the higher state.

There is, however, one important factor that is generally overlooked by modern writers on the subject. This relates to the development of certain moral qualities that form a precondition for any form of spiritual enlightenment. There is a general tendency in this age to overlook or belittle this important aspect of spiritual effort. The idea prevailing in the minds of many people is that certain simple techniques are necessary to attain an entry into the occult and the supernatural, and that all one has to do is to practice these techniques to achieve the goal. Some even believe that there are backdoor methods—magical formulas, *mantras*, or charms that can lend enhanced potency to spiritual disciplines and practices—so that one can even expect automatic results. Unfortunately those who think in these terms seldom look around to see what has been the harvest of such methods. Have even a handful out of the millions of seekers who practice such disciplines been able to effect a breakthrough and reach the promised goal? If not, on what practical results achieved in modern times does their belief rest?

■ *For thousands of years there has been a belief in the efficacy of* mantras. *It is held by exponents of Mantra-Yoga that the sounds proceeding from the pronunciation of certain letters and words or combinations of words in a certain way create peculiar vibrations by their reasonance that greatly enhance the chances of success in Yoga, attainment of psychic gifts, healing powers, and other siddhis. What is your opinion about it?*

It is true, of course, that sound vibrations can have physical effects. It is well known, for instance, that lines of marching soldiers crossing a bridge can cause tremors in the structure, and that loud talking in high mountains may start a snow avalanche. But mere recitation of a *mantra* can have no effect on the acceleration of the evolutionary processes if it is not accompanied by the other disciplines and virtues that form a necessary element of spiritual progress. A *mantra* or a *mandala*, when accepted and acted upon with faith, may serve the purpose of creating a mental condition favorable to success. We know from experience that a placebo, or chemically inert pill, given to a patient by a doctor with the suggestion that it is a specific medicine for the ailment may prove effective in curing the disease.

But the active agent is not the *mantra* or the pill, but the faith of the subject and belief in its efficacy. It is mind working upon itself. The same thing also happens in the case of quack medicines, spells, and charms. The potency of a *mantra*, a quack medicine, a talisman or a charm, rests mainly on suggestion or autosuggestion in the subject himself. The power of suggestion grows when there is a mass application of the *mantra* or the quack remedy. This can even take the form of mass hysteria. The power of dictators rests on their skill to make appropriate use of words and suggestions. When Hitler spoke, millions upon millions of people were stirred to their depths by what he said, until mass hysteria swept over the whole of Germany. The infected crowds realized the gravity of their mistake only when it was too late. Even intellectuals caught the infection and were swept off their feet in spite of themselves, deluded into the belief that they belonged to a master race destined for rulership. The *mantra* specialist does the same sort of thing. He tells a follower, often in privacy, that he is on the way to becoming one of the elite if he practices his methods. Since this often accords with the disciple's own wishful thinking, he readily believes what is said, and for this confirmation reveres the teacher all the more.

The same thing has happened and will continue to happen in the case of mass movements that are not grounded in truth. No artificial method that does not conform to the demands of nature can ever succeed in leading seekers to higher states of consciousness. It is tragic that sometimes even intelligent seekers are carried away by the false thinking of the time and do not stop to reflect how a radical transformation in consciousness can come about by the chanting of a few words, or by any other artificial device, when no such method has ever been successful in changing a blockhead into an intellectual. Whether transcendental experience betokens communion with the Deity or ascension to Cosmic Consciousness, it is evident that a man-made artifice or talisman can have no place in the natural order of things. The use of *mantras* or spells denotes a stage of mental development where the critical faculty has not been developed sufficiently to understand that the operation of inviolable laws of nature cannot be affected by charismatic performances.

I am emphatic on this point, because I feel that the employment of *mantras* or any other kind of chicanery to cheat nature, whether in the material or spiritual world, can only lead to failure and disappointment. Recourse simply to *mantras* or quick ways to attainment of spiritual objectives must, in the long run, lead to a state of mind that depends on magical and miraculous windfalls rather than on one's own hard efforts. Such a frame of mind, especially among young people today, is fatal for the progress of any country, both in the material and spiritual fields. It is a softening of the brain, an unmistakable sign of degeneration and decay. A person or group that loses confidence in itself and depends upon the intercession or psychic power of another to gain a sublime goal is obviously seeking a way of escape from the storm and stress of the battle of life, a state of mind that never brought glory to any individual or nation.

The one great lesson that history teaches is that only those nations that depended on their own initiative, effort, or strength of arms rose to ascendency. Can we attribute the position of eminence occupied by any nation at present—as, for instance, the United States, Russia, Japan—or the freedom gained by others—for example, India—to the potency of a *mantra* or a talisman or to a combination of sounds, causing certain kinds of vibrations in the astral world? Did any individual or family rise to prominence, wealth, power, or wisdom by any such means? If not, how can one expect these methods to bring one nearer to God? The mere idea that it can happen is a negation of Divine Justice and a mockery of law and order in the spiritual world.

But the belief in the success of *mantras* as a shortcut to higher states of consciousness is as firmly rooted as the faith in *mantras* and charms for power and wealth. In order to show the false nature of this belief it is necessary to lay due emphasis on the role played by the brain and the body of man to achieve altered states of consciousness and to make this knowledge available to the masses.

There can be no doubt about the fact that every state of consciousness is reflected in the brain, in the body, and even in the bloodstream. We all know the physical influence exercised by our emotions such as anger, fear, depression, worry, and passion. They cause such marked reactions on the organism that the physiological changes can even be measured objectively. Unshakable evidence, dating back to prehistoric times, shows that altered states of consciousness experienced in ecstasy and mystical trance also have an effect on the body. Ecstasy in the cases of Saint Teresa and Sri Ramakrishna was attended by a rigidity of the body, coldness, diminished breathing and heart action, and other such symptoms as accompany a swoon. In such cases there is complete or partial insensibility to all outward impressions. In other cases, however, although the body is undoubtedly affected, the effect does not express itself in the extreme form of a cataleptic condition or loss of sensibility. In other cases the sensory channels continue to function, but the impressions they bring create now a different world. The surrounding scene assumes a sublime aspect, as if viewed through a more elevated channel of

perception, investing every object perceived with a glory that
was never observed before.

We need not enter here into the issue whether this alteration
in consciousness is brought about by the mind or the body,
whether initially the change occurs in the brain or is due to an
impulse from the latter that causes changes in the organ of
thought. It is sufficient to state here that the two are so closely
interdependent that the change in one involves a change in the
other. For a *mantra* to be effective it is therefore necessary that
its repetition, whether done silently or audibly, should lead to
changes in both the components. If this does not happen it
means that the vision evoked has no basis in reality and can only
be a product of suggestion.

If a *mantra* has the potentiality to cause organic changes in
brain matter, leading to expanded states of consciousness, then
it must also have the capacity to cure mental and nervous disorders by effecting appropriate changes in the brain and nerve
cells that cause the maladies. It should also be able then to
erase the difference in the intellectual stature of different people,
make a simpleton into a genius or a fool into a sage. But is there
even one specialist who can help rid humanity of the growing
menace of mental ailments simply by the use of a *mantra*, or
any other talisman of this nature, or grant the boon of intelligence or even common sense to the myriads of mentally deficient or underdeveloped unfortunates of our time? If not, what
faulty thinking makes us put blind faith in charismatic methods
for gaining transcendental states of consciousness or approach
to Divinity, involving a complete metamorphosis of personality,
when no such method has ever been able to correct even one
single mental illness out of the host of psychic plagues that
cause suffering to millions?

There are hundreds of *mantras* in use at present, and the initi-
ator of every one of them claims the highest efficacy for it. That

some people feel stimulated, and even have visionary experiences of some sort, provides no evidence for the efficacy of a particular *mantra* or a set of *mantras* for gaining access to higher dimensions of consciousness. The simple-minded Tibetan used to turn a prayer wheel in the vain hope that so many million repetitions of the *mantra* would bring him relief from worldly ills and procure salvation in the other world. Mere recitation of a *mantra* without devout meditation, cultivation of cardinal virtues, and purity of heart can never lead to enlightenment. The realm of the spirit is as much subject to law as the physical world.

The very method of initiation of a *mantra* conveys to the initiate a suggestion that merely by repeated chanting of some sounds he can gain the desired goal by the grace of the Guru. Yet are *mantras* of a utility in passing examinations, in gaining knowledge of science and arts, in winning athletic prowess, in gaining votes in an election, in achieving success in any profession, or in arresting old age, or in any one of the countless spheres of human activity in which man would like to be helped and rescued from the drudgery of pain? If not, are we to believe that God-realization can be attained without hard and systematic toil merely by the chanting of a few words? Surely a most comic and paradoxical position for the Lord of Creation, since for every other objective He has ordained right thinking and hard labor as the means to attainment, however trivial, transient, or unimportant the goal may be; but strangely enough, according to the advocates of the *mantra* tradition, made a singular exception in His own case. Can one seriously believe that the same Creator, who has bound the universe in inviolable law, would prescribe no more than simple mechanical chanting of a string of words to win to Him, or the whole creation of which He is Lord?

If success in spiritual enterprise, resulting in the development of mystical consciousness, were as easy to attain as is confidently predicted by many teachers of Yoga, then the mystery that still surrounds the numinous would have ceased to exist long ago. But for most people the transcendental realm is as inscrutable and mysterious now as it ever was in the past. Those who promise speedy and easy results are either themselves ignorant about the arduous nature of the task or are deliberately misrepresenting the issue for reasons of their own.

A glance at the life stories of Yoga saints, mystics, and seers of the past show that all of them, without exception, had certain strongly marked mental characteristics present often from birth, and most of them gave evidence of high ethical standards throughout their lives. The most prominent of these traits was their love of truth, devotion, hard-fought battles for perfection, love for their fellow beings, altruism, and a sense of detachment from the world. Many modern teachers of Yoga slur over these essential traits in order not to have any moral strings attached to their systems. By doing so they repudiate all the scriptural authority of the past. In no genuine system of spiritual discipline was ethical teaching divorced from the practices and observances undertaken to gain religious experience, as has been done now under the mistaken idea that it is the methods and not the ordering of one's life in conformity to certain ideals and principles that is the real key to success in every spiritual and religious enterprise.

■ *At present there are many teachers of Yoga and many ashrams for instruction in this science. Since Yoga and other systems of religious discipline stimulate kundalini, leading to a heightening of the evolutionary processes, does this mean that all those who undertake these disciplines will attain to expanded states of consciousness?*

This depends on a number of factors, for instance, the earnestness of the seeker, his physical and mental attributes, good bodily and mental health, heredity, noble traits of character, benevolent disposition, and other factors about which we are at present in the dark but which will come to light in the future. The methods and practices employed and the mental attitude maintained during the course of training can also contribute to the success of the undertaking. Those who evince perseverance, zeal, love and devotion for the sublime enterprise have a much greater chance of speedy success than those who lack these qualifications and virtues.

But many teachers of Yoga claim universal efficacy for their methods. They assert that everybody can benefit from them, irrespective of their mode of life, habits, and occupations. The point therefore arises whether there can be universally effective methods that can help seekers realize their objectives or dreams? Before discussing the point, the first thing to be decided is what exactly is the dream or ideal in the mind of those who submit themselves to mental or religious disciplines of this kind.

An expanded state of consciousness or vision of the Deity is, generally speaking, the main aim before many seekers who take to religious or mental disciplines, but there are also many people who seek psychic gifts, occult powers, success in worldly enterprises, enhanced mental efficiency, physical health, or inner peace and happiness by the use of these methods. There are also some who are not very clear about their own aims. They take to the disciplines when they see large crowds doing so, more in response to the herd instinct than to any clearly defined objective in their mind.

Both in India and elsewhere the ordinary class of Yoga teachers are not very clear about the exact condition to which their methods can lead. The boons generally promised are self-unfoldment, God-realization, superconsciousness, mental or physical efficiency, peace of mind, or paranormal gifts. Many of the teachers, particularly in the West, guarantee peace of mind, creative intelligence, physical and mental efficiency, and inner happiness. A higher dimension of consciousness or the experience of Divinity is seldom brought into the picture. The utmost that is said is that one can attain to self-awareness or gain control over his subconscious. It is true that God-realization or Cosmic Consciousness might be sometimes implied in such methods, but what is openly propagated is their ability to confer mundane benefits, health, peace of mind, inner happiness, and greater mental efficiency with their methods.

■ *Why do you make these distinctions? Aren't physical and mental health, intellectual and artistic talent, inner peace and happiness a part of the harvest brought by illumination? Don't the enlightened gain these benefits side by side with a higher state of consciousness?*

They certainly do, but I am making the distinction purposely to show that illumination is the fundamental target of Yoga and every healthy form of religious discipline, and that all other benefits and merits accrue from it. Etymologically "Yoga" means union of the individual soul with the Universal Spirit, and all great authorities on the science have laid emphasis on this aspect of the discipline. There is a gulf of difference between a teacher of Yoga and an enlightened man. The former may be well versed in some of the techniques employed but has no personal experience of the ultimate goal. He may have personally practiced the various disciplines—Shat-Karma, Asana, Pranayama, Dharana, and Dhyana—and studied a mass of literature on the subject, but still remained entirely unaware of the extraordinary state to which true Yoga finally leads.

On account of this great difference, there is sometimes no concordance between what the unenlightened Yoga teacher pre-
scribes for his disciple and what the illumined adept says. The
former, who fails to rise beyond the dry disciplines and mechanical techniques, has nothing except the models or method and
practice before his eye, while the enlightened one, who soars beyond the body, mind, and intellect into a world of eternal light
and life, develops a far better grasp of the virtues and mental
attributes that are necessary in one who tries to soar to the same
ethereal height. This is the main reason why the writings or dis-
courses of great sages like Sri Ramakrishna, Abhinava Gupta,
Ramanuja, Kabir, and others turn again and again to the cultivation of ethical virtues and lofty traits of character as the essential prerequisites in one who aspires to Divine Consciousness. In
fact, all the leading luminaries of India, including the Adi Shankaracharya himself, have given a secondary place to the mechanical disciplines of Yoga as compared to the lofty mental and
moral attributes necessary for success in a spiritual undertaking.

The ordinary teachers of Yoga, inexperienced in this stupendous transformation of limited human consciousness into a cosmic state of being, confine their attention to the worldly benefits
that can be derived from Yoga. This is not at all a new direction
taken by the exponents of this hoary science in the present age.
There have been countless Yogis, even in the past, who, defeated
in the bid to attain a higher state of consciousness, concentrated
on worldly objectives. They attracted even larger crowds of disciples, allured by promises of occult powers and worldly gains.
The works of some of them are still extant, condemned by suc-
cessive generations of enlightened adepts as the futile attempts
of deluded men to put to mundane use a lofty science designed
for a sublime aim.

History repeats itself. The misinterpretation and abuse of
Yoga that ultimately led to darkness and degeneration in India

and reduced it to a state of servitude for centuries have now extended their sphere of influence to the West and will cause the same conditions as they once did in India. The distaste for the battle of life, addiction to drugs, and wanderlust that characterized the degenerate form of Yoga in India, will characterize it in Europe, America, and other places also. When once the lofty goal of a spiritual discipline is lost, obstructed, or deliberately distorted by everyone who employs it for his own purpose and aim, imprinting his individual stamp and form to the teaching he is imparting, then no power can save the science from deteriorating and degenerating to the position of a salable commodity, which anyone thinks he can buy for a price.

How can you expect a harmonious development of the human personality when professional teachers of spiritual disciplines outbid each other in their attempt to prescribe cheap and easy methods of mind culture without first stressing the need for the cultivation of those lofty traits of character in their disciples without which entry to higher states of consciousness is impossible? We know very well that moral reformation has been the main target of the teachings of all great spiritual luminaries of the past. It would be the height of unwisdom to suppose that any modern teachers understand the secrets of spiritual transformation better or are more enlightened than Buddha or Lao Tse or Christ or Vyasa (the author of the Bhagavad-Gita), and have better knowledge of the methods that can lead to illumination than these widely acknowledged masters of spiritual science.

As I have already stressed, the true aim of Yoga and other healthy spiritual disciplines is an expanded state of consciousness, a glorious consummation that raises man from the world of death and darkness to the transcendental world of eternal life and light. When, instead of placing this sublime goal before the searching eyes of the would-be aspirants, we substitute worldly success, mental efficiency, and quietude, in a highly competitive world, it means that we veil the real, natural goal from their eyes, shut out a glorious future that is the natural heritage of every man and woman, and supplant it with inferior worldly objectives with which they are already over-occupied. When we do this, we kill the natural incentive for noble thought and deed in individuals, replacing it with ignoble aims and objectives, like the race for excessive power and wealth. Do we not already see the ominous signs of the havoc wrought by these base impulses in the present hate-torn and envy-ridden world, threatened with disaster without parallel in history? Whatever the method or discipline used, any system of Yoga or any method of religious discipline that does not lay sufficient stress on the cultivation of cardinal virtues can never lead to illumination, for the reason that development of moral attributes is as necessary for self-unfoldment as teething is for the normal growth of a child.

■ Aren't mental peace, efficiency, and creativeness of paramount importance for the purpose of a happy and successful worldly life? If so, what is the harm if some spiritual teachers prescribe methods to achieve these aims?

Yes, they are most essential for a happy life. The point is, however, whether a happy individual life is the only target that has to be kept in view in order to fulfill the purpose of human life. The attainment of lasting happiness, immortal life, and exhaust-less wealth has been a constant thirst of the human mind, and time after time countless men and women in the past devoted their lives and resources to this ceaseless quest. The search for the philosophers' stone and the Elixir of Immortality provided the lifelong occupation of many highly intelligent and persevering minds. Even a saint like Thomas Acquinas evinced keen interest in the transmutation of metals, while Roger Bacon included in his studies the art of prolongation of life by means of alchemy. But did anything of substantial value ever emerge from the efforts of countless individuals in this direction? Neither the Elixir of Life nor the philosophers' stone ever became possible.

In our own day there are hundreds upon hundreds of Yogis, occultists, spiritual teachers, mediums, Sufi masters, and others who prescribe various methods for the development of the worldly qualities mentioned, each of them speaking highly of his own method, with testimonials from crowds of admirers and followers; but has the world become in any way wiser, richer, calmer, or happier by it? Why this has not happened is because there is a definite evolutionary target prescribed for human beings. If this target is not kept constantly in view as the ultimate goal of our exercises and disciplines, and if the mind is directed toward the achievement of objectives and aims that fall far short of it, then our endeavor cannot really fructify, for the reason that the exclusion of the real purpose of a natural process can never lead to healthy results. It is because of this that all the founders of great religions, prophets and seers, prescribed union with Brahman, God, Ishvara, Allah, Jehovah, a Celestial Being, or unfoldment of Self as the supreme aim of life, alloting a subsidiary place to other physical and mental objectives.

It is the sun that illumines the world and enables life in all its innumerable forms to grow and thrive on earth, and not its reflections in the lakes, rivers, and oceans. In the same way, it is the expansion of consciousness of the ascent toward the beatific state, the source of all peace, happiness, and creativity that, like the sun, nourishes and illumines our mind and helps these attributes to grow. This, therefore, should be the target of all our efforts and not the mere acquisition of physical or mental gifts, because the shutting out of the sun from our sight implies turning away from the illuminating source of all to plunge into the gloom of uncertainty and error, and in that case we could never know in which direction our way lies. This is the reason why none of the existing systems of mental training and discipline has been able to play a decisive role in resolving the present confusion prevailing about the destiny of man. Once this goal is ascertained and accepted, methods for its achievement and the acquisition of other mental attributes—peace, happiness, creativity—will follow as a matter of course, supported by all the resources of science. There will then exist no need for occult sects and creeds, esoteric systems, doctrines, or secret practices and disciplines, each bearing the stamp of a separate self-styled Yogi, Master, adept or expert, but the whole enterprise will take the form of a scientifically oriented religious undertaking for all mankind. And all the methods, disciplines, and practices, both in the East and the West, will, after investigation and sifting, form the nucleus of the methodology applied to this new branch of knowledge, by far the most important of all the existing branches taken together.

■ *Do you mean that it is only when we become fully aware of our spiritual destination that we can attain to true inner peace, happiness, and finer gifts of the mind?*

In a sense this is right. The awareness of the destination implies also an awareness of the paths leading to it. Ignorance about the destination implies also ignorance about the path. The choice of the path lies with us, but only when the knowledge of the destination is complete can we choose the best and safest route ourselves. This, in turn, will make us aware of the mode of life we have to follow to make our voyage safe.

The whole structure of human society—its politics, religion, jurisprudence, social construction, education—is based on the assumption that man is the final object of creation, and there is as yet no universal recognition of the fact that he is in a state of transition, not only mentally but also organically toward a sublime model on which civilized man based his pictures of angels, gods, and other celestial beings. It is the evolutionary impulse in the human brain that has brought heaven and its empyrean denizens to life in the imagination of man. But there is little inkling of it at the moment even in the minds of the most erudite. It is this fatal gap in our knowledge about the evolutionary target of mankind that is at the root of the present highly explosive situation of the modern world.

"What are we here for?" "What is the purpose of all this stir and bustle around us?" are questions which we must be in a position to answer in order to be able to decide what role we are expected to play in order to make the best use of our life. Without an answer to these questions we can only flounder in the dark, ignorant of the direction we must take, ignorant of our own transgressions and mistakes, and also ignorant of the way in which they can be rectified. In such a milieu, efforts made for the acquisition of certain physical and mental gifts or inner peace can never be wholly successful, whatever the methods employed, for the simple reason that in the absence of the knowledge of the goal, inadvertent disregard of principles necessary to attain it can never lead to a happy consummation. This again is the reason for the present unsettled and unsatisfactory condition of the world.

■ *What is your opinion about saintliness? Are saints an ornament to society? If so, what purpose do they serve?*

Before answering, it would perhaps be better to define the term saintliness. In general usage, the word "saint" denotes a holy man, eminent in virtue, who has turned wholly to God and practices religious disciplines for spiritual ends.

It is easy to infer that such a man would be an ornament to society, provided he does not withdraw himself to such an extent as to be dead to human sentiment, and indifferent to the hopes and aspirations of his fellow beings, provided also that he is not over-conscious of his own piety and virtue, and freely associates himself in altruistic actions with his fellow beings for the common good.

Unfortunately saintliness also provides a venue for egotism and pride. A saint who believes that piety and self-restraint raise him to a position of superiority to other human beings, and in this belief arrogates to himself the position of a Guru, a healer of souls, or a hierarch, is not an ornament and can even be a menace for society. He falls in stature below those who, with no pretensions to piety, humbly extend their help to the greatest extent possible to those who need it. Among worldly men and women there are individuals who, without knowing it, lead more sublime and nobler lives than some of those who have the reputation of being saints, living away from the world and its turmoil, and therefore cut off from the area of fellow feeling and humanity. And among even saints there are individuals whose overweening ego and pride nullify all the other virtues that they possess.

In the context of religious teachings, where God is the object to be attained and purity and holiness are the essential ingredients of character in one who sets himself on the path, withdrawal from the world, celibacy, monasticism, and austerity might, with justice, be considered as fitting attributes. But once we accept that religious striving is, in fact, a method for the acceleration of evolutionary processes and that the ultimate aim of saintliness and piety is to gain a higher state of consciousness, then the whole issue assumes a different color altogether. Then the place of precedence should naturally be occupied by those who lead exemplary lives in the world of men, participating nobly in the battle of life, sharing the burdens, the joys, and the sorrows of their fellow beings, and acting in a manner friendly and beneficial to all, so that by their contribution they leave a better and richer world behind them. Such an ideal of life has been beautifully expressed by Kabira, the famous Indian mystic, in these words: "When you took birth, O Kabira, the world made merry and you cried [the first cry of the newborn and the jubilation of kinsfolk on the birth of a male child]. Act now in a manner that you are jubilant when you pass away, while the whole world grieves [at your death]."

When religion becomes entirely an end in itself and the world fades away from sight, then the mind may fall prey to obsession and eccentricity. In fact an abnormal state of mind is a clearly marked symptom of extreme asceticism. It could not be otherwise, for complete withdrawal from the battle of life cannot but have unfavorable psychological reactions because of the violation of the natural instincts involved in such a mode of conduct and behavior. Of all the many different religions, there can be no single infallible system, for *kundalini* may even be aroused in individuals outside the pale of organized religions. This is amply corroborated by the fact that spontaneous forms of mystical ecstasy occur even in those who are not tied to any religious belief and have not undergone any specific religious discipline.

■ *If kundalini is the basic mechanism responsible for all varieties of genuine religious experience, then why are there so many different esoteric practices and disciplines and so many* divergent forms of Yoga, such as *Jnana, Karma, Raja, Hatha,* and the like?

The varied nature of religious practices and disciplines and the existence of different systems of Yoga corroborate my views about *kundalini*. When we admit that all religious experience, in order to be genuine, must have its base in the biological structure of the body, we are then at once faced with the question as to what this biological base can be. The only way to answer this question is to assume an organic potentiality in the human body that, under certain circumstances, creates those conditions of the brain and nervous system in which the experience becomes possible.

Without a biological base we are left with the alternative that the mystical condition is hallucinatory, with no relationship to the organism as a whole. If the experience is purely hallucinatory, then there is no need to probe into the body-mind relationship that is responsible for it, and in that case, there is also no need to discuss the potency or diversity of the various methods and disciplines employed, for the reason that each individual can use his own method for inducing a hallucination of his choice.

But keeping in view the fact that all methods of religious discipline, all esoteric practices, and all schools of Yoga have some specific exercises and disciplines in common, as, for instance, concentration, devotional worship or prayer, constant thought of the Divine, and cultivation of certain virtues such as self-restraint, truthfulness, purity of mind, benevolence, and the like, it is obvious that this systemization has a particular influence on the body and mind complex to create the states of consciousness responsible for ecstasy. If this were not so, the various practices and disciplines would be so widely dissimilar as to have nothing in common. But a close study of the numerous practices, exercises, and disciplines in vogue from times immemorial, both in the East and the West, shows that they are all variations of the few basic principles of which concentrated mental application, devotion, and purity of mind and body are the chief.

That all these practices impinge on some specific organic system in the individual naturally follows. A whole group of exercises and disciplines, all containing certain basic features in common, could not come into existence in different lands and at different periods of time, unless the very constitution of the human body, or, to be more precise, of the human brain, demanded such a systematic training to induce certain extraordinary states of mind and consciousness. The fact that there are diverse systems of Yoga, and also widely divergent religious methods and disciplines, with a certain similarity in essentials in either case, leads to the obvious conclusion that this variation is partly due to the difference in climate and culture of the people by whom the disciplines were designed, the period of time when this was done, and partly to the difference in the constitution and temperament of the individuals to whom they were applied.

This is at once clear from even a cursory study of the Hatha-Yoga and Raja-Yoga systems of religious discipline. Hatha-Yoga concentrates on physical positions, while Raja-Yoga is concerned with spiritual development. Hatha-Yoga embodies certain exercises and practices, some of which are not only revolting but even dangerous for a sensitive system. Many of the Hatha-Yoga exercises are pure gambles with death, and it is no wonder that during a strenuous course of training there are many cases of loss of life, sanity, or health among the sadhakas or aspirants. The Hatha Yogis themselves acknowledge the superiority of Raja-Yoga and it is held that after success in Hatha-Yoga, the exercises of Raja-Yoga are necessary for the highest *samadhi*. This is clearly admitted in the Hatha Yoga Pradipika, well-known treatise on Hatha form of Yoga. "Those Yogis who while practicing

Hatha-Yoga have no perception of Raja-Yoga," it says (4.69), "I consider them to be void of the fruit of their labor." The reason for this is obvious. The ultimate aim of every form of Yoga is transformation of consciousness. Mere bodily exercises and practices, even done to perfection for prolonged periods, can bear no harvest until the mind is harnessed with Raja-Yoga disciplines to enable unfettered consciousness, watered by the ambrosia of *kundalini*, to soar to transhuman levels of inexpressible happiness and peace.

As can be readily understood, *kundalini*, the perennially active evolutionary mechanism, is not uniformly effective in all men and women, but varies enormously from one end of the scale to the other, depending on the vital organs and physical and mental traits of different individuals. There is a vast range of difference between the evolutionary level of one individual as compared to that of another, in the same way that there are vast differences in the intellectual levels of various people. This furnishes us with a clue to the mystery as to why one system of exercises is more effective in some cases than in others. There are many forms of Yoga, in addition to Hatha and Raja. For example, Karma-Yoga is concerned with good actions, Jnana-Yoga with knowledge, Bhakti-Yoga with devotion.

It is idle to expect that an illiterate rustic can ever grasp the real significance of Jnana-Yoga, that is, cognition of the Reality through intellectual discrimination, however much one may try to explain it to him, let alone command enough intellectual acumen to put it into practice. Similarly Bhakti-Yoga is primarily intended for such individuals in whom devotional sentiments preponderate. Raja-Yoga becomes effective in cases where mental and physical discipline is necessary to bring the body to that state of evolutionary preparedness where a leap into a higher dimension of consciousness becomes possible. Extreme austerity and penance, though clearly abnormal and unhealthy forms of self-discipline, might well be needed in some cases of physical or mental recalcitrance, where moderate disciplines can prove of no avail. Since the various systems of mental and bodily discipline employed for gaining transcendence were devised centuries, perhaps even millennia ago, and during this interval of time humanity has taken a more forward leap in evolutionary ascent, the time is now ripe for a thorough overhauling of all such practices and exercises, in order to discover what will best suit mankind at its present intellectual and aesthetic level.

■ *Would it be right to infer from what you say that human beings are so diversely constituted in this respect that some need extremely stringent, some stringent, some moderate, and some easy methods to arouse kundalini and that it is not practicable to prescribe one uniform discipline applicable to all cases?*

How can it be otherwise when some people are at the top of the evolutionary ascent and some at the base? How can you equate a simpleton with an intellectual in the race for enlightenment? The latter has already traversed part of the way. From the evolutionary point of view, a man of genius is already close to the boundary line from which the enlightened state begins. Only little effort is needed for him to step across the line. In fact, the mystical tendencies and experiences of men like Plato, Newton, Einstein, Wordsworth, Tennyson, and others arose because of this extremely thin barrier between the consciousness of a genius and the perennially illumined sage. This is also the reason why high intellects sometimes exhibit mystical traits.

The avowal of Pascal about his profound ecstatic experience in which he says, "joy, joy, joy and tears of joy," recorded in his own hand and found stitched up in his doublet after his death, is not an isolated instance of spontaneous spiritual unfoldment, but only one of countless such occurrences among the intellectual hierarchy of mankind. The reason why there are not many confessions of this type is because in some cases the experience was not understood and classified; in other cases it was not recorded or disclosed, out of reluctance to make private matters publicly known, or out of fear of ridicule of friends and colleagues. The last-mentioned reason applies especially in the case of scholars and savants of repute. The exercises of Jnana-Yoga are sometimes sufficient, in such cases of intellectual maturity, to induce higher states of consciousness even without entering into a regular course of Yoga training or any other religious discipline. This is also the reason why large numbers of people, even in Europe and America, who have no knowledge of *kundalini* and have never practiced Yoga in their lives, have had spontaneous flashes of illumination and even ecstatic experiences. Not being able to ascribe any rational explanation to these extraordinary conditions, they often remained mystified, a prey to doubts and uncertainty, sometimes all their lives.

"There is no need to practice extreme asceticism or the retention of breath for attaining to Sahaja (oneness with Universal Consciousness)," says Lalleshwari. "Merely by wishing it you may gain the door to freedom, and, dissolved [into the ocean of life] as salt is dissolved in water, you can taste the Inexpressible."

5   The Problem of Miracles and the Paranormal

■ *Why do people so persistently associate miraculous powers and paranormal faculties with enlightenment? This attitude has been invariably seen from the remote past, yet we find that the founders of some major faiths openly denounced miracle-mongering. In India, the belief is common that the exhibition of psychic powers is a great obstacle in the part of God-realization.*

The main reason for the association of miraculous powers with enlightenment lies in the fact that from the earliest epochs magic has been closely associated with religion. In the most primitive societies, in fact, no distinction was made between magic and faith. The deities worshipped, whether in the form of idols, natural objects, or forces of nature, were all invested with magical powers, and the various practices and disciplines undertaken for worshipping and propitiating them were often regarded as methods for the acquisition of magical properties. The shaman, the witch doctor, the oracle, or the magician were regarded with awe and fear on account of their magical skill and treated as channels for approach to the hidden intelligent forces of nature. With the advancement of civilization, even after the shaman, the oracle, and the magician had been replaced by the seer, the prophet, the mystic, and the Yogi, the primitive practice of investing a holy man with supernatural powers continued with but slight modifications unaltered to this day.

The miraculous power ascribed for ages by primitives to the shaman and the witch doctor never worked to emancipate the people from the crushing weight of superstition, ignorance, illiteracy, contagious diseases, obnoxious social customs, and tyrannical political systems. Liberation eventually came only through advance in knowledge or through intermingling with more advanced groups and populations whose unfettered intellect had already lightened the load of these evils. The reason why primitives and the semicivilized set such store by supernatural agencies and charismatic delivery from difficulties was rooted in the very natural position that, helpless against the relentless forces of nature and bodily afflictions, they knew of no other way to escape from these otherwise unavoidable evils.

If you look carefully and dispassionately, you will find that belief in the miraculous powers of saints, mystics, and Yogis is like the mirage of an alluring oasis in a burning desert. Though it appears most attractive and invigorating to a traveler famished with hunger and parched with thirst, it always remains beyond his reach until he falls exhausted through vain pursuit of the enchanting vision still before his eyes. The same is true of people who, in pursuit of worldly ambition or freedom from some evil that dogs their steps, look around for a miraculous way to solve their problems.

There is hardly a single individual among thousands who does not have a problem that weighs on his mind and that he has not been able to solve, despite all his efforts. Some lack wealth, some beauty, some children, some health, and many peace of mind. Some want more power and prestige, others more influence. Some long for a deeply cherished object, others for the love of an adored being. Some fear an inveterate enemy, the anger of an injured person, or the displeasure of a ruler, and some wish to rid themselves of habits or other nuisances that continually harass them. In short, almost everybody has a problem on his mind from which he ardently seeks a way of escape. Some also have a burning desire to solve the riddle of their own being, but they lack the strength of purpose to achieve success in the endeavor and therefore look for someone else to serve as a prop in the undertaking.

The human mind has an innate thirst for everlasting life and the vigor of youth. There is no picture so heart-rending as that of emaciated age, the drooping figure and wrinkled face, sunken eyes and sagging mouth, the fire of youth extinguished, trembling and shaking, a brooding, senile mind living in the faded past, waiting apprehensively day and night for the approach of death. For many people, the thought of enfeebled age and the oblivion of death is unbearable, and they fervently desire to find a way to prevent the dreaded climax. The promises held out by exponents of certain esoteric spiritual disciplines seem to them to provide the only way to avoid the catastrophe. Laboring under pressure of problems, fears and frailties, countless people look around for an easy way of escape, and captivated by alluring accounts of miraculous occurrences contained in scriptures and books about the occult, search for some adept to help them out of their difficulties. The primary reason why many seekers after the Divine show such humility and pay such homage to spiritual men, ascetics, and Yogis, rests on the fact that they generally consider them to be supernormal and expect a miraculous intercession from them to meet their own spiritual or temporal needs. Such people clearly exhibit a lack of self-confidence and a dependence on others for the solution. This weak-kneed attitude in itself constitutes a great stumbling block in the path of self-realization, as the supreme prize of Cosmic Consciousness demands courage, self-reliance, and other manly qualities in those who would strive for it. There are few, indeed, who seek the company of spiritual teachers merely for the sake of enlightenment.

It is no wonder, then, that the miracle-working Yogi exercises a tremendous influence and draws enormous crowds of admirers and followers. This has also been the position in the past. Even men of intelligence sometimes fall prey to the delusion that a state of enlightenment necessarily denotes a state of power over the elements and the occult forces of nature.

A moment's reflection will show the fallacious nature of such an assumption. Were the power of performing miracles or producing psychic phenomena amenable to human control, and were there any adepts possessing full command over such extraordinary powers at their will and choice, there should have developed a regular science of the occult and the miraculous long ago, as demonstrable and as capable of universal application as material science is in our own time. But this is not the case. On the contrary, we find that it was only when talented men repudiated the supernatural and broke the bonds of superstition forged by religion that the human mind was able to overcome a host of disabilities imposed by nature and find relief from diverse ills and evils to attain the present state of material prosperity and comfort. Yet while enjoying the warm glow of countless amenities provided by intellect and science, some credulous seekers after enlightenment still cherish hopes of a miraculous breakthrough to paranormal levels of consciousness merely by the powers of some adept, forgetful of the strict laws of causality that govern every event in the universe and to which they owe all the amenities and joys of life.

If we allow our fancy to dwell on the past and contemplate the superstitious primitive with a strong belief in the supernatural and the miraculous, we find little sign of improvement in his miserable condition wrought by magical means. Surveying the whole subsequent span of history, do we see at any time— even during the lives of the greatest seers and prophets—unmistakable signs of widespread amelioration of the human condition? Has there been any mitigation of the tyranny of nature over man, any relief for the sick, the downtrodden, and the weak, brought about by the miraculous power of any saint, seer, or magician? True, there have been isolated miracles, some paranormal phenomena, and small-scale magical feats, often intermingled with fraud and self-deception, but no widespread or significant victories over nature. Whatever great and lasting improvements have been effected have all been due to the power of intellect applied by talented men and women, believing in their own efforts and skill, without reliance on the supernatural or the occult. Even the powers of healing, displayed by a few adepts in the past and exhibited by some psychics today, are not possible of universal application. They are isolated faculties that never made the art of healing richer by suggesting ways for a more correct diagnosis and a more effective cure of disease, applicable to all and sundry, irrespective of time and place. For every patient cured by the touch of a healer there are thousands who recover from disease by the normal methods of medical treatment.

Mankind depends, as it has in the past and will continue to do in the future, upon intellect for battling with the problems of life, for understanding the causes of disease and prescribing the appropriate remedies for them. Psychic healing, paranormal phenomena, and miraculous acts, to become firmly established and universal, first require knowledge of the forces involved. Ascription of miraculous powers and magical control over the elements to saints or spiritual men is based on primitive superstition, because the real basis of spiritual experience and psychic faculties still continues to be a mystery. All these phenomena provide a very important subject for study and investigation. So long, however, as they continue to be unpredictable and erratic, it would be tragic if, instead of solving their problems in the natural way, people were to wait for miraculous occurrences to overcome them.

Space does not permit me to describe the horrible methods sometimes used by psychic healers among primitive and backward people to exorcise imaginary evil spirits from the emaciated bodies of patients in the grip of organic diseases, needing a regular course of treatment for cure. It is not difficult to imagine what aggravation or prolongation of agony and loss of life must be caused by the employment of rough and crude methods, when there is no understanding of the cause or prognosis of a malady. Nor is it difficult to visualize how many failures, resulting in torture or death, there can be for every successful cure that is widely publicized. At present there is no greater hurdle to the right understanding of the true spiritual goal and the success of any undertaking to that end, than the superstitions and irrational beliefs that still persist in the mind of man.

A dogmatic approach to the science of healing, however, can be as retrogressive as dogmatism in religion or other branches of secular knowledge. What is needed is study and experiment until the basic laws or forces responsible for them are known. Unconventional methods of treatment, such as faith cure, psychic healing, nature cure, diet cure, earth cure, acupuncture, and the like, that have a confirmative history behind them, ought not to be rejected because they do not fall in line with the orthodox methods in use at present, for the simple reason that our current systems had a similar beginning from crude and self-devised methods of healers and physicians of the past, before they were knit into a regular science, capable of universal application. The same open-minded and broad approach ought to be adopted in the case of methods of healing that are now classified as unconventional or unscientific.

■ *What can be said about the extraordinary psychic exhibitions of mediums, sensitives, occultists, Yogis, and others in the past and that even now can be witnessed somewhere almost daily? There have been, as we know, instances of prophets, mystics, and Yoga adepts who have healed the sick, made water flow from rocks, raised the dead, made spirits to materialize themselves, walked on water, visited distant places in the astral body, and worked other miracles that were surprising in the extreme.*

I don't deny that certain gifted individuals, mystics, saints, or adepts have sometimes provided such evidence. But there are limits to their displays. What is considered in one case to be due to an extrasensory faculty may in another be classed as a miracle. For instance, a dowser, divining a source of water with the use of his rod or pendulum, is thought to be in possession of a special sense, but a saint, who strikes the ground with his staff and has his followers discover a pure stream of water, is more likely to be credited with having worked a miracle. One very important point that has to be kept in view when considering miraculous events and psychic phenomena is that in many cases it is not the possessor of the power but the power itself that is the master of the situation. The exhibition of these powers has almost always been erratic. Those who demonstrated them had little control over the manifestations. It is a well-known fact that many spiritualist mediums and sensitives have been found guilty of trickery at one time or another. When the power did not manifest itself before an expectant audience, the medium resorted to artifice to save his reputation.

A striking instance of this kind showed not only how credulous a crowd can be in regard to the supernatural, but also to what extremes imposture can be practiced in this domain. I allude to the news that flashed around the world a few years back that an embryo in the womb of its mother in Indonesia was able to recite the Quran in a manner distinctly audible to the hearers! Thousands surged forward to attest the authenticity of the miracle, but eventually the fraud was exposed. In a more primitive environment the imposture might well have remained undetected, surviving as an example of a miracluous occurrence like many recounted in the religious literature of mankind.

Again, admitting that some individuals do possess paranormal faculties of various kinds, let us consider what has been their impact on the historical development of mankind. What part have they played in the social, political, material, or even spiritual progress of the race? Most of the founders of major faiths emphatically repudiated miracles and condemned their use. They occupy an insignificant position in the most popular and authoritative scriptures of India, as for instance, the Bhagavad-Gita and the Upanishads. There is no historical record to establish that miracles enriched any human being, nor is there the least evidence to show that any individuals rose to be kings, ministers, generals, or millionaires by such means. Nor has any great scholar, thinker, scientist, painter, or musician ever attributed his extraordinary talent to them. It is surprising, therefore, that so many people remain ever on the lookout for a miracle-worker to help them, or at least to satisfy their curiosity about the supernatural.

We know that modern science completely discredits miracles and supernatural occurrences, and the reason is not difficult to discover. The Renaissance found Europe in the grip of religious dogma, superstition, and a cramped intellect, with irrational belief in black magic, witchcraft, spells, and charms. The masses relied on the efficacy of amulets, talismans, potions, and magic for fighting even virulent diseases and bodily deformations. Science eventually triumphed with rational theories and methods, and what was considered impossible of human achievement—

except through magic or a miracle, as, for instance, flying—became possible with knowledge of material laws. How far we have succeeded is shown by the amazing efficacy of modern drugs for controlling deadly diseases and plagues, and the marvels of painless surgery. Most people who now submit calmly to the extirpation of a malignant tumor would find it difficult to imagine the horror of a major operation performed centuries ago.

Had those superstitious beliefs and dogmas continued to sway the intellects of the rising generations, the present era of reason might never have dawned at all. The world would have continued to be in the grip of pestilence, famine, natural calamities, ignorance, and poverty. Those who seek miraculous solutions for difficulties or ailments seldom realize that some of the common gadgets they use daily would be no less than magical objects in medieval times.

It is indeed paradoxical that while enlightened Indians are trying to liberate their country from the tentacles of superstition and false beliefs, imaginative westerners are carrying to their own lands those same deceptive ideas and erroneous beliefs that have already done incalculable harm to the East! Instead of drawing the pure, fresh water from the springhead of the ancient seers and sages, they take back the muddy and contaminated ideas of the charlatans, and the result of this has been that some modern youth have regressed to a primitive level in their knowledge and even in their concepts about the spiritual and the Divine. Many thousands of them gullibly swallow embellished accounts about the magical properties of *mantras*, and stories about the alleged miraculous ability of spiritual teachers to induce higher consciousness in others merely by a glance or an act of will. It is incredible that people readily ingest stories of this kind, while all the while conscious of the fact that no saint or adept ever undertook or could accomplish the far easier feat of upraising the mental level of Mongoloids, cretins, idiots, blockheads, and others of that category, to the level of intelligence of average human beings, a most humane undertaking that could bring the light of understanding to millions.

Perhaps the greatest evil that stems from uncritical belief in the miraculous and the magical is self-deception. There can be no more glaring proof of this than the plight of the thousands of seekers after the Divine who, abandoning their careers and homes, come to India and other Eastern countries for instantaneous self-realization, often returning home as empty-handed as they came. They present a most pitiable picture to all sober-minded people, who realize the hopelessness of their quest. Had the miracles they seek any real existence, or magic any real potency, the holy men who indulge in self-advertising would have no need to take such pains to attract crowds of followers or gratify them with instantaneous *mantras* or magically produced gifts. It would save them a lot of labor and worry and be very much in their own interest if they were to work a miracle on themselves, to cure their morbid thirst for adulation and applause, and act in accordance with scriptural injunctions to confine their activities to the teaching of spiritual knowledge and wisdom. They would then leave a legacy of Truth, immune from the onslaughts of time, like the immortal teachings of the illuminati in the past.

The thousands of mediums, psychics, and sensitives in Europe and America, with all their exhibitions, have not been able to arrest in the least the materialistic tendencies gaining ground every day. Their amazing feats, even in Russia, have made no dent in the skeptical attitude of the Communist intellectuals. What resistance, therefore, can a few *mantra* specialists and miracle-workers put up against the rising tide of skepticism and disbelief that threatens to engulf the whole of mankind? They do not help to strengthen but, by the hollow nature of their methods, tend to scatter the force of spirituality and truth. They do not seem to realize this, nor do those who admire their ways. There are well-intentioned men who believe that whatever the nature and the substance of a spiritual movement, it should be allowed to grow and spread to combat the gathering forces of irreligion and disbelief. These good men often fail to see that an untruth, masquerading as truth, does greater damage to a holy cause, when its falsity is exposed, than can be done by the antagonism of fair-minded opponents.

■ *When it is well known to Christians, Buddhists, Muslims, and Zionists that the great founders of their faiths, their prophets and seers, aligned a certain specific path for them, emphasized the cultivation of certain cardinal virtues, and laid the utmost stress on the surrender to and love of God as the shortest way to emancipation, from where has this hunt for miracles and magical formulas come? And why are so many people attracted to this misleading path?*

There are several factors responsible for this state of affairs. The most important is that religion has become isolated from recent phenomenal progress in other branches of knowledge, and has been kept at a distance, as if it is something untouchable or obnoxious with which the well-informed should not be concerned. The very application of the term "secular" to politics, social affairs, education, and the like is an indication that in almost all spheres of man's worldly life, religion is considered to be an outcast. This is an issue of supreme importance. If religion is the outcome of an innate tendency in man, its exclusion from his temporal sphere cannot but be unhealthy and unfavorable to his well-being to a dangerous extent.

The present ignorance about the true facts, and the prevalence of wrong and delusive notions concerning the Divine and the miraculous, owe their origin to this inane apathy toward the spiritual life and the unhealthy isolation of religion from the other spheres of human activity and knowledge. There is no other study in which there is such uncertainty, conflict, and confusion as in the realm of faith, and this state of affairs at the present evolutionary level of mankind is most prejudicial both to its safety and its sanity.

Another reason for this serious lack of knowledge about the spiritual world lies in the very constitution of the various major faiths of mankind. The doctrines contained in a book or a set of books have to be accepted without question as the infallible dictates of revelation. This leaves little scope for the exercise of reason. Even if there is some flexibility, as, for instance, in the six systems of Hindu philosophy, the touchstone upon which the deductions of reason are to be tested is again a revealed scripture, in this case the Vedas.

Stagnation is anathema to nature. The emphasis of some of the organized churches on the unalterable and impregnable nature of scriptural lore is not in accordance with the progressive aims of nature and cannot survive the onslaught of time. The consequence of this fallacious viewpoint—the fruit of human vanity, thinking too highly of itself and its doctrinal beliefs and ideas—has been that the ancient faiths, one and all, now face a crisis. Many of their dissatisfied adherents are turning to other faiths and creeds to satisfy the deep-rooted urge for spiritual knowledge. This has, in turn, led to an unprecedented increase in the number of cults, and to the paradoxical situation that even the failures in other spheres of life find ready crowds waiting to listen to them in the amphitheater of faith, treating them as their spiritual guides or gurus. They forget the obvious truth that the founders of their faith, whose teachings they now ignore, were among the greatest spiritual prodigies ever born.

The rush for instant enlightenment is so precipitous that no one has time or inclination to ascertain the actual goal for which the religious thirst exists in man, and whether this goal can actually be attained by the new and cheap methods prescribed by the pseudo gurus. The main factor responsible is ignorance about the truth of religion. In their eagerness for quick results, people often forget the difficult nature of the task, and hoping against hope, turn to the purveyors of faith who promise rich dividends with very little investment, in the belief that one of them, at least, might reveal a shortcut to the goal.

■ *If the power of working miracles is detracted, in what respect then would the enlightened rise above the normal level of human beings? How can we distinguish them from the average run of mortals?*

Let us first consider the question whether it is reasonable to assume that ascension to a higher state of consciousness must be attended by miraculous powers, or, in other words, control over the subtle forces of nature not possible for ordinary human beings. We know very well that humankind has attained to its present lofty intellectual stature by a gradual process of evolution, and although we do not yet know all the mechanisms, we do know that we find no evidence that this evolutionary climb was attended by supernatural manifestations, or that man came into possession of any paranormal faculties side by side with the rise in his intellect.

Since the whole process has been ruled by strict biological laws, how can we then reasonably expect that in the now succeeding evolutionary climb the previous order would be set aside and miraculous or supernatural manifestations attend the process, endowing the enlightened or fully evolved individuals with magical powers never before possessed? The fact that there are still-hidden forces of nature, exhibited in psi phenomena, and that the future man might be able to control these forces at his will, does not imply that they form part and parcel of biological evolution as it has occurred so far or that they can at any stage intervene to give a twist to the laws governing the same. Future man may attain to a stature where he can master intelligent forces of nature in the same way that he has attained mastery over the physical forces with his intellect. But even this mastery would not allow a radical departure from biological laws—only a better understanding of the forces responsible for the phenomenon of life. The accumulation of more precise data about *kundalini*—and the study of the conditions attending enlightenment—should make it easy not only for scholars but also for laymen to recognize one who has attained to a higher state of consciousness.

As a rule, he should be characterized by four exceptional attributes, namely, genius, psychic talents, lofty traits of character, and an expanded state of consciousness. By the term "psychic talents" I do not mean miraculous or magical powers, but higher mental faculties, such as clairvoyance, precognition, highly developed intuition, and the like. According to Indian authorities, the most remarkable characteristic of enlightenment is *jnana* or the outflow of perennial wisdom. This is a fragrance that is designed to perfume the whole blooming garden of humanity. *Jnana*, in the present-day language of science, is the attainment and the expression of that priceless knowledge that is essential for the evolutionary progress of mankind and that is as true now as it would be after millennia. It is intended to guide the footsteps of the race on the winding and tortuous path of evolution. This is a province about which the intellect can provide no information because of its inability to look into the future both near and far.

■ *But we have instances of mediums whose performances border on the magical and miraculous, who can cause spirit materializations, who can make objects move without any contact, or provide evidence of strange formations, as for example ectoplasm, or who can produce other kinds of physical phenomena. If ordinary mediums and sensitives are able to display these powers, why can't the enlightened also exhibit them by virtue of their contact with the higher planes of consciousness?*

Some psychic mediums can produce phenomena that are hard to duplicate by any other class of men, but the psychic powers exercised by the enlightened are of a more refined and far-reaching character. They have a universal value for all mankind. There is no doubt that some sensitives and mediums have done immense service to the cause of knowledge and science by bringing the still unexplored levels of mind sharply to the notice of intelligent people with their extraordinary demonstrations. Some of them have been great healers, some honored interpreters of religious truths, and some channels for the exhibition of the phenomena of materialization, telekinesis, and so forth.

There is also no gainsaying the fact that some of them devoted their lives and their extraordinary faculties purely to the service of knowledge without any idea of personal gain. Though we fail to understand it at the moment, there must be some purpose in the appearance of men and women of this category from time to time. They have been a persistent feature of human existence from prehistoric times. It can be possible that they are intended by nature to serve the very useful purpose of drawing attention to the planes of creation hidden from the sight of man because of the poverty of his sensual equipment. They excite curiosity to a high degree and thereby serve as means to draw attention of investigations to the phenomena until the laws governing the forces responsible for them are known.

It has to be stressed that the phenomena produced by mediums and sensitives, though they now command the credence of a large percentage of scientists, have not yet been finally accepted as proved and established beyond dispute. One reason why many scholars are hesitant in according general recognition to this category of psychic phenomena is that so many mediums, at one time or another, were found guilty of trickery or fraud. Then, too, the occurrences have been, as a rule, erratic. Some mediums resorted to deception because they did not have complete control over the forces that manifested themselves through them. They often lived completely under their sway.

Mediums sometimes lie insensible or in semitrance condition when the phenomena occur, presenting a pathetic picture of helplessness to the investigators or audiences who witness their performances. No truly enlightened individual would like to be in such a position. For a voluntary control of these forces and for their universal application in the service of future man, free from uncertainty and capriciousness, a further advance in the evolutionary stature of the race is necessary. The enlightened man or woman of the future is likely to win over these forces with the application of the higher channel of perception—the Third Eye—that will develop in him in the same way that modern man uses his intellect for the solution of material problems.

Spinoza's criticism of miracles—that they cannot happen because they violate the order of nature, and thus God would be contradicting Himself, since nature is fixed and changeless—presupposes complete knowledge of natural laws and the forces working in the universe. This is far from the actual position. We still do not know what laws rule matter at the basic levels of creation. Hume's argument that "no testimony could establish a miracle unless its falsehood would be more miraculous than the alleged miracle itself" contains its own refutation: The condition laid down for acceptance of miracles is impossible of

fulfillment, for a "miracle" is at present beyond human understanding and control.

Thomas Huxley's approach is more rational when he says,
"Any seeming violation of the laws of nature would be investigated by science and its existence would simply extend our view
of nature." In the case of miracles, psi faculties and spiritualist
phenomena, we deal with intelligent forces beyond the perceptual range of our senses. We call them miracles and supernormal
displays because these fine stratas of the cosmos are hidden from
our view. Michael Scriven's remark, "Give me a good ESP
experiment—goodbye physics," expressing the fear that irrefutable empirical evidence of psi phenomena would invalidate our
present-day knowledge of physics, is not well grounded. Empirical certitude gained about the existence of finer forces of nature,
manifested in paranormal displays, cannot nullify our experience
of the gross physical world. It would simply lead to a healthy
expansion of our views about the universe as a lawful whole.

The phenomenon of life is itself a visible, conclusive proof of
the interdependence and mutual harmony of the physical and
superphysical laws. The corporeal and incorporeal parts of all
organic structures are so closely allied and function in such uni-
son, it is as if they were drawing their nourishment from the
same root. Our wishful thinking or narrow-mindedness drives
us either to place too much reliance on the miraculous and the
supernatural, drawing satisfaction from the thought that we
might be the fortunate recipients of such grace, or to reject them
altogether. Whereas, the more rational attitude would be to
investigate them thoroughly and sympathetically, without undue
bias toward either side.

There is no comparison between the experiments I propose
to validate *kundalini* and those designed to investigate psychi-
cal and paranormal phenomena. The latter have been under
scientific study now for about a century without providing

reproducible-at-will conclusive evidence about the validity of many of the occurrences observed. Nor have they led to the identification of the forces involved. This poverty of results is incredible, considering that hundreds of able men and women, including distinguished scientists, have been investigating these phenomena for many years. They have not even made an appreciable dent in the skeptical armor of orthodox science.

■ *If, as you say, there is hardly any possibility of gaining control over the intelligent forces, manifested in psi phenomena, then it means that the time and energy expended at present in the investigation of the occurrences would not lead to any tangible results, and mankind will continue to remain as much in ignorance about the intelligences responsible for them as it is now?*

I do not say that the time and labor spent on this research has brought no fruitful results. What I mean is that the exploration of paranormal phenomena is not likely to yield the harvest expected of it by some investigating agencies. For instance, there is no possibility that the nature of the forces at the bottom of these displays can be ascertained with the methods employed at present. If we have not been able to fathom the mystery of normal consciousness, how can we reasonably expect to solve the riddle of its paranormal exhibitions? The issue of the control of these forces can only arise when their nature and the laws under which they work are well known. So long as we are not in possession of this knowledge there can be no possibility of gaining control over them.

But some other definite advantages are always there. The investigation could lead to a better understanding of the phenomena, resulting in the breaking down of the hard barriers

erected by orthodox science against the acceptance of the existence of spiritual and intelligent powers in the universe, and to
the recognition of consciousness as an independent, ever-existing
cosmic substance. The investigation can also result in the discovery of the biological factors peculiar to the individuals who
exhibit psi faculties, which would mean a tremendous advance
in the knowledge about the subject. Such research can lead to
further additions to our existing knowledge about mind and consciousness. If the exhibitions are not witnessed simply to satisfy
idle curiosity or to gain material benefits by supernormal means,
they can also provide spiritual solace and conviction of other-
worldly existence and the powers of the spirit.

We have no satisfactory explanation for the inexplicable
phenomenon of consciousness. Every materialistic system of philosophy is an attempt to sidetrack it. Every fact that we know
about the universe is channeled through our mind, and we have
no real knowledge of anything that is outside or beyond it. A
child often ignores what it cannot explain or assigns fantastic
reasons for it. The primitive mind invariably resorted to the
supernatural and the miraculous for the explanation of natural
phenomena. The reason of the primitive was completely satisfied
with the irrational explanations offered by elders and priests, who
themselves believed in what they said, having heard or learned
it from their predecessors. This frame of mind of the savage is an
enigma to us, since we are not constituted that way. But when
we recall our childhood and succeed in evoking a correct picture
of it, we then come to notice the difference between mature and
childish ways of thought. We then remember that many stories
and anecdotes that now appear incredible and even nonsensical
seemed perfectly natural and correct during childhood. This
change is as much due to experience as to the development of
the rational faculty in the majority of people. But there are individuals who continue to think as children to the end of their

lives! This is especially true of their ideas about the miraculous and the supernatural. The superearthly or the magical has such a fascination for some minds that they can believe almost anything on the subject. They at once lend credence to every sensational episode related to them, however fantastic and unbelievable it might be.

The reason why millions of people become enthusiastic followers of irrational and bizarre creeds and cults, and often defend even absurd dogmas and beliefs associated with them, lies in the existence of an infantile streak in them concerning the Supramundane. We see this frailty exhibited in the irrational religious beliefs of many otherwise highly intelligent people. Blind faith or uncritical belief is always hungry for marvels. People like to hear positive stories supporting their fantastic beliefs, even if these stories are incredible. The result is that their critical faculty, alert in all other matters, almost ceases to function in this particular direction. To a uniformly rational mind it seems almost impossible that there should be people so credulous toward alleged occurrences of the supernatural as to lend credence to accounts that are palpably untrue and entirely unbelievable. To a large extent this can well be due to a paralysis of the reasoning faculty caused by the long domination of organized religion, banning the exercise of critical intellect in respect of the spiritual and the Divine. We also encounter this partial atrophy of the critical faculty among modern youth in their search for enlightenment, when they discard time-honored methods in favor of much-publicized, time-serving techniques that promise sure ways to self-knowledge for a price!

A striking example of this is the avidity with which fantastic stories about the alleged miracles performed by certain Gurus and Yoga adepts are accepted uncritically even by the educated. It is noteworthy that there are more anecdotes about the miraculous powers of Indian fakirs and Yogis from the pens of western

writers than from Indian scholars! For many decades the notori-
ous magical rope trick of fakirs provided an exciting theme for
western writers. But since the interest in the subject has dwindled, no one comes forward to say that he had witnessed such a
performance. Why? Have the fakirs who performed this magical
trick vanished from the land? One reason for this might be that
as soon as somebody makes a claim of having witnessed such a
feat, he would be asked to substantiate his statement by producing the performance. But if somebody in America recounts a
similar episode about a miracle-working Yogi in the depths of
the Himalayas, the story is often swallowed, and no demand for
proof is raised because of the sheer distance involved.

Western writers frequently come to India with their minds
full of ideas about adepts and Yogis capable of performing
miraculous feats. A mind already possessed by a fixed idea often
falls easy prey to imposture and trickery, or is deluded by its own
obsessions. People of this type implicitly believe what they are
told without inquiry and investigation, or even themselves con-
jure up hallucinatory pictures of what they expect or are asked
to see. The famous rope trick was known to be an illusion and
was cited in scriptures as an illustration of the fallibility of mind
and senses, as in the Vedantic simile about the rope that might
appear to be a snake in darkness or uncertain light.

The stories and life histories of saints and Yogis written by
their disciples especially abound in miraculous anecdotes and
tales. "Spiritual teachers do not fly in the air," says a Persian
proverb. "It is their disciples who make them fly." In fact, it is
the flavor of the supernatural and the miraculous that endears
such narratives to a large class of readers of the occult.

There is no mention of miracles in the descriptions of the
supreme experience in the principal Upanishads, the fountain-
head of metaphysical and spiritual thought in India. Buddha
condemned the performance of miracles as a sin. The Bhagavad-

Gita, most popular of India's scriptures, does not even mention the word "miracle" when defining Yoga. Its whole teaching is directed to the proper ordering of life and the cultivation of virtues necessary for the attainment of higher states of consciousness. Patanjali, the famous author of Yoga-Sutras, treats the desire for psychic gifts as an obstruction in the attainment of self-knowledge or realization. Guru Nanak, founder of the Sikh religion, is emphatic that miracles imply a negation of God. Mohammed also discredited the working of miracles. In fact, there is a common agreement among the spiritually minded in India that the power to perform miracles, even if developed during the course of Yoga practices, is more in the nature of a pitfall on the path, or a test of the fidelity of the seeker, rather than a means to help him onward on the divine quest.

Not one of the great modern Indian saints and sages, such as Sri Ramakrishna, Maharshi Ramana, Sri Aurobindo, Swami Dayananda, or Swami Sivananda, endorse the exhibition of psychic gifts or the working of miracles, even if endowed with such powers. It is, therefore, strange how the alleged possession of psychic gifts and miraculous powers exercises such a fascination over a certain class of modern spiritual seekers. This must be due to a desire to find an easy way of escape from the stern demands of a strictly causal world. A moment's reflection, however, shows the futility of such a hope. Most of us live surrounded by the innumerable amenities provided by science, the product of man's unceasing search for the secrets of nature, and the bountiful harvest of his tireless efforts to verify empirically the postulates of the intellect.

Out of countless discoveries, inventions, creations, and innovations, during the last five thousand years, is there a single verifiable achievement or event of history that had a miraculous origin? Aside from legend, is there a single war, calamity, famine, or epidemic that was averted or miraculously controlled?

What weakness in our mental constitution, then, drives us to lend credence to fabulous stories and to hope against hope that by extensive search or study we can find a hidden secret, a marvelous individual, or a miraculous occurrence that can lead to our material uplift or spiritual unfoldment?

It is said that Sri Ramakrishna, one of the greatest spiritual geniuses of our time, wept bitterly when he visited a famine-stricken area and saw the horrible suffering of the people. He exhorted the Rani, who had accompanied him there, to help them with relief. If miracles have any substance and are permissible on a large scale, could he not have removed their dreadful suffering with but an act of will?

There is no great spiritual teacher in India, either ancient or modern, who advocates miracle-mongering or the employment of magical methods to win to transcendental states of consciousness. Their whole emphasis has been on leading a good life. If the claims made in the Yoga-Sutras of Patanjali, the HathaYoga Pradipika, and other manuals on Yoga were to be accepted literally, then all the achievements by science could be possible through the instrumentality of individual willpower or the merest wish of one single adept.

"As a result of Samyama [combined *dharana, dhyana,* and *samadhi*] there arises the intuitive knowledge of Cosmic spaces," says Patanjali in the Yoga-Sutras (iii-26), and again (iii-27), "By Samyama upon the moon there arises knowledge of the arrangement of the stars." Yet again he writes (iii-29), "By Samyama upon the Chakra of the navel there arises knowledge of the arrangement of body." The point that arises here is this: Whether knowledge of the cosmic spaces or of the stars or the physiology of the human body was brought up to its present high level of progress by the efforts of ascetics and Yogis, with *pranayama* and other allied practices, or by normal men and women with the proper application of their intellect and powers of observation, and with a spirit of dedication to science.

The confusion between what can be achieved by the intellect and what is the utility of the higher channels of perception is at the root of many misconceptions that have been current in the past and continue to this day. But if Yoga is to be understood in a broader sense, namely, as a system of culture for the mind and body to win wider and still wider states of consciousness, talent, and genius by the conditioning of the brain and the nervous system, then Samyama—that is, prolonged concentration and absorption—is certainly the method employed for gathering knowledge, ascertaining new facts, and making fresh discoveries in all spheres of thought.

It is important to distinguish between the powers claimed by Yogis and the miracles and psychic phenomena of mediums and others. Hindu religious geniuses and the originators of the science of Yoga practice, by observation of the forces released in their own bodies with prolonged meditation or other religious practices, developed the concept of *kundalini*, and it still remains the most valuable theory to meet the facts of higher consciousness. In contrast, miracles and all other kinds of paranormal phenomena are not amenable to one uniform interpretation, and as a rule are erratic and unpredictable. They have been instrumental in drawing people away from true spiritual development or scientific advance. During the many centuries since the time of the early religious geniuses and devout practitioners of Yoga, there has been so much exaggeration and confusion, such growth of legends and superstitions, that even the reality of *kundalini* and higher consciousness have become fabulous. It is now time to attempt a synthesis that can reinstate the fact of *kundalini* in a manner acceptable to modern knowledge and science.

In ancient India, China, Arabia, Greece, and Rome, inveterate skeptics, who discredited miraculous feats and supernatural occurrences, flourished side by side with the credulous, who believed in them implicitly. This position still exists. Psychic phenomena are so rare, erratic, and undependable, and the men and women who exhibit them so much in the grip of mysterious forces and so little able to exercise voluntary control over them, that the investigation itself becomes a will-o'-the-wisp chase which never yields a tangible clue.

In the case of experiments connected with *kundalini*, the object is not the pursuit of mysterious uncanny forces to establish the validity of strange and bizarre occurrences, but rather it is the investigation of a biological phenomenon as clearly observable and measurable as the physiological processes occurring, say, at pregnancy. The only reason why there is such solid incredulity among the learned about the outcome of such experiments is that the phenomenon is so rare. This is probably the first time the awakening of *kundalini* has been represented in its psychological effect on consciousness and also in its bearing on the biological organization of man, thus exhibiting the continuity of the psychosomatic relationship that results in the manifestation of consciousness in normal and supernormal states. The popular present-day concepts about *kundalini*, based on the traditional presentation of it, ignore the biological aspect altogether, treating it as a superearthly, if not supernatural, force dormant in the human body, which, when aroused, suddenly creates amazing alterations in the personality and leads to miraculous or divine powers.

The wrong assumption that the phenomenon of *kundalini* is purely psychic in nature and has no base in the organic structure of the body or the gross material of earth, has been one of the main stumbling blocks in understanding and establishing its real nature. For that matter, this assumption applies to any inexplicable phenomenon connected with religion and the occult.

The dogmatic attitude of various faiths has added not a little to these obstacles, as almost all religious doctrines firmly seal the frontier connecting the spirit with the body. They never allowed reason to probe into the mysterious happenings that differentiate religious experiences from the causal events of the earth.

The belief in the incompatibility of the psyche and soma is so rife that few individuals see any possibility of finding a common basis. From the early philosophers, like Kapila in India, to men like Descartes, there has been an attempt to draw a sharp, ineffaceable line between the spirit and the body, often ignoring the fact that if the spirit is nonspatial and nondimensional, and the body material—subject to the play of space and time—there must be some sort of a connecting link between the two. With all this background and the prevalent notions about religion and mystical experience, the idea that the body continues to play a decisive role in the development of higher states of consciousness and the ecstatic trance of the mystic can only appear novel and maybe even fantastic.

This especially holds true for the cynics, to whom man is only a bundle of passions and desires with no promise of a total change from his present state toward a sublime and glorious life in the future. For them, he is what he has always been and will continue to be what he is now.

The variety of beliefs and philosophical speculations leaves very little room for the acceptance of the view that mystical experience and spiritual phenomena—of the kind witnessed from time immemorial to the present day—have as close a relation to the organic structure of the men and women who exhibit them as normal consciousness has to the average human body and brain. This relationship can be clearly demonstrated with the experiments I propose. They can be repeated on men and women from different countries and of different faiths and beliefs. The biological reactions on the awakening of *kundalini* would invariably be the same, with possible slight modifications due to different temperaments or physical and mental constitutions of the individuals. In every case of a successful awakening, leading to a transformation of consciousness, the accelerated metabolic processes, the flow of the reproductive secretions, and the circulation of transmuted sex energy, would be definitely noticed for varying lengths of time.

Once the biological processes are started, they continue to work in a rhythmical fashion in the same way they function in the normal course. The uncertainty and unreliability that attend abnormal psychic phenomena is entirely absent in this case, because the change is an organic one, as regular and systematic as organic changes are, and not a passing phenomenon outside one's reckoning and power of minute observation. The only point of similarity between the two lies in the fact that the force that sets the transformative processes in operation on the arousal of *kundalini,* and that which seems to revel in weird, grotesque, or childlike acts of a poltergeist, or indulge in pranks of materialization and telekinesis in psychic phenomena, is equally mysterious in origin. However, the awakening of *kundalini,* properly accomplished, is a healthy development instead of a freakish exhibition involving perplexity from start to finish.

■ *But why is it that in spite of the fact that the ideas expressed about* kundalini *provide a workable hypothesis for the forces involved in the obscure phenomena of genius, mediumistic gifts, and mystical experiences, the scientific community does not immediately welcome the proposal for investigation and proceed with experiments to prove or disprove the truth of your statements?*

The question is probably based on the assumption that the

moment a new plausible explanation is provided for any inexplicable phenomenon of nature the world will at once welcome it. Even a cursory knowledge of human nature and events of the past make it amply clear that whenever a new and unexpected line of thought or action was presented, there was always more resistance than readiness to grasp or act on it. We know what trials awaited the great teachers and founders of new faiths and the pioneers of science. Most of them had to suffer hardships and tribulations, and in earlier times even faced death in their endeavors to make the Truth known. It is still an inexplicable paradox why people are more ready to accept false and sometimes even downright harmful views and doctrines and to adopt the superficial or foolish customs and habits of others than to assimilate true teachings and emulate noble traits of character in their search for reality and true happiness. Did not opposition to his ideas in the initial stages force even Max Planck to exclaim that only the progeny would understand him?

Another strongly marked trait in human nature is the tenacity with which people hold to a point of view to which they are wedded. This fantastic state of mind is sometimes so intractable that most people in this category either lack the understanding to know the truth or refuse to see it, even when the falsity or absurdity of their own point of view is conclusively demonstrated. This applies not only to the common masses, but also to the well-informed. The number of people who keep their minds open to the inflow of fresh ideas and concepts is comparatively limited.

However rational and valuable the disclosures about *kundalini* might be, therefore, it is idle to expect that they will be readily accepted or cause an immediate change in thinking. Indeed, it would be more prudent to anticipate a good deal of opposition and resistance on account of the present dogmatic attitude of both the staunch adherents of major faiths and the orthodox expounders of modern science. It is also possible that in this advanced era of specialization and division of knowledge, the opposition encountered might even be more pronounced than in the past. This is because a unilateral development of thought is almost always prejudicial to a balanced outlook on life and its infinitely varied expression or spheres of activity. Thus an expert in military strategy thinks in terms of war and destruction, an astronomer in terms of stars and their movements, a physician in terms of disease and death, or a psychiatrist in terms of mental abnormality and disorder, rather than of life as a whole. Only those who have explored interdisciplinary research and have gone beyond specialization can display the same deep understanding and value for all branches of knowledge or points of view. In the light of these facts, it would be too much to expect that my revaluation of the ancient doctrine of *kundalini*—as providing a workable key to some of the hitherto unsolved mysteries of mind—would meet an immediate ready response from the numerous specialized branches of knowledge, ideologies and faiths into which mankind stands divided at present.

■ *If this is the position, it means that the mere comprehension of the idea would take an indefinite period of time. What do you have to say of its acceptance and the subsequent empirical investigation by competent scholars and men of science?*

Yes, that obviously is the normal position. But the manifestations of *kundalini* are so varied and operative in so many departments of human life that, according to my thinking, their impact will soon be felt in various avenues of knowledge, especially in some of the branches dealing with mind and consciousness. These would be in the spheres of insanity, extrasensory perception, altered states of consciousness, mind-expanding drugs, hypnotism, mediumistic phenomena, genius, and the like.

The repercussions of this impact will immediately be reflected in allied departments of study and generate the ripples in thought that will ultimately lead to a thorough investigation of the whole phenomenon sooner than one might expect. If the effects of *kundalini* were confined to but one exclusive field of study, say mystical experience, the process of acceptance and verification would be far more protracted, and it would take a long time indeed before the ideas would be accepted and become an integral part of our knowledge. But here we are dealing with a biological force that is operative in many directions connected with the evolution and survival of mankind; so once its spheres of activity are known and understood, a sudden unfoldment of new facts, whether brought about by accident or deliberate investigation, would bring the whole subject prominently before the rank and file of science.

Nature does not rest content with merely the calculated efforts of human minds. Most of the great discoveries in the past were stimulated by flashes of sudden insight in those whose brains were already in tune. But for this extraordinary phenomenon, human progress could never have been possible. We do not know precisely what causes, besides persistent labor and concentrated thought, work to bring about this highly intuitive and responsive state of mind, but we are certainly in no doubt about the gratuitous and unpredictable nature of the phenomenon. The insights about *kundalini* that I have gained fall within the sphere of such occurrences. Only I had to experience its varied expressions on myself, and this resulted in a long period of suffering and suspense. Just as this insight did not come about by a calculated effort on my part, in the same way the verification of my assertions can also occur with similar insights gained by others, specializing in different departments connected with the manifestation of *kundalini*. It is also possible that events or circumstances may combine forcefully to draw the attention of some investigators to a symptom or characteristic peculiar to *kundalini*, leading to the recognition of this mighty biological force in a flash of intuition similar to mine.

We are aware that there are sometimes certain inborn mental defects, as with congenital physical disabilities. But we have no overall view that relates such misfortunes to a general evolutionary pattern, rather than to random biology and chemistry in the context of behaviorist philosophy. This does not mean that there is no explanation or that such things will continue to be clothed in doubt and obscurity until the end of time. Certain phenomena of nature, for which fantastic mystical explanations were furnished by the primitive mind—eclipses, for instance—awaited solutions pending attainment of a certain level of intelligence and scientific discovery. When this was reached, the explanation was found without difficulty. There is nothing more necessary for a seeker after Truth, whether a common man or a scholar, than to keep his mind open for new possibilities in the solution of the mysteries of nature. Unfortunately, some individuals, mistakenly overconfident of their own learning and experience, have been instrumental in spreading erroneous notions about thought and consciousness, tending to create the impression that some of the still-unsolved problems of insanity, genius, psychic gifts—and other exceptional and paranormal faculties of mind—*have been long since settled.*

There is a great divergence of opinion among the learned about the nature of consciousness and its relationship to the physical organism. Some of them, still wrongly laboring under the weight of materialistic thought of the nineteenth century, continue to move in the same old groove, unable to accept the position that consciousness is an incorporeal energy, totally beyond the reach of our sensual equipment. They still believe that the brain is the generator of consciousness or, at least, that the two are inseparable, instead of realizing that the former is a frail and delicate instrument of an Almighty Cosmic Intelligence that expresses itself in both limited and unlimited awareness *through* it.

The postulate of *kundalini*, therefore, has to pass many hurdles before it is likely to win acceptance. The domain of the superconscious and the paranormal is still a subject of dispute, and much confusion prevails about the nature of transcendental experience and the possibilities of true psychic phenomena. The present position with regard to consciousness can be compared with justice to the position of various physical sciences, such as astronomy, chemistry, physics, physiology, medicine, and the like, in pre-Renaissance days. There has to occur a breakthrough in the pedantic and confused mass of scholastic speculation about consciousness. When this breakthrough occurs, even the first fleeting glimpses of the reality underlying it will be sufficient to cause a complete revolution in the current conceptions about life and bring into prominence the glorious future destined for man.

6 Science and *Kundalini*

■ *How can investigation into* kundalini *lead to an under-standing of the phenomena of mystical expreience, genius and psychic faculties?*

All these three extraordinary manifestations of consciousness—for which science as yet has no explanation—depend mainly upon the transformation of *prana* or bioenergy. The size and shape of the brain remains the same, but there do occur subtle changes in the biological composition of the cells and the nerve fibrils, although we have no means to determine these changes at present. There is also no doubt that a new activity starts in the brain, due to the opening of a normally closed chamber to the influx of a fine biochemical essence, rising from the reproductive region through the spinal cord. This extract serves as nourishment for the highly enhanced activity leading to an expanded state of consciousness. The activity—stimulated by a new and more potent form of bioenergy drawn by the nerves from all parts of the body—flows through the spinal conduit in a luminous stream to cause the explosion in consciousness characteristic of the arousal of the serpent power and its ascent to the *sahasrara*, alle-gorically depicted as the thousand-petalled lotus in the brain.

Subjectively, this flow of the essences, culled from the repro-ductive organs, can be distinctly felt in the space behind the palate, from the middle point to the root of the tongue. It pours into the cranium in an ambrosial stream so exquisitely pleasurable that even the rapture of love pales into insignificance when compared to it. At the same time the erstwhile, narrow-orbited consciousness is perceived spreading on all sides in ever-widening waves of lustrous being, until it attains the dimensions of an effulgent, unbounded ocean of awareness in which the wonder-struck ego, with only a faint recollection of its corporeal existence, appears like a dim and distant piece of floating corkwood, bobbing up and down, lost in the immensity of the expanse surrounding it.

The descriptions contained in the Tantras and other treatises on Hatha-Yoga, about "the dripping ambrosia on the union of Shakti with Shiva," in actual fact denote the streaming of the reproductive secretions into the brain, on the opening of the central canal with the arousal of the *kundalini* power. These secretions are then drawn up as if a powerful suction is applied from above to the nerves lining the *kanda* (the triangular space below the navel) and the *muladhara cakra* (the plexus close to the anal opening). This marks the initiation of a new organic activity in the body in which the brain, the nervous system, and the reproductive organs are the main participants in an effort to fashion the whole system to a new awareness beyond the normal limits of human consciousness.

I am making these statements from full personal experience of this extraordinary psychophysiological development. This upward flow of the reproductive essences into the cranium through the spinal canal is definitely somatic in nature. The body of the awakened individual develops a new biological function and a new form of awareness with a supersensory channel of cognition. The constant perception of luminosity, both within and without, which is an invariable characteristic of higher consciousness, makes the observing soul appear as if attired in a sheath of light.

This is why, in the ancient books on Yoga and on spiritual lore, mention is made of the development of a "shining body" or a "diamond body" or a "perfect body" as an auxiliary to enlightenment. It is a clear indication of awakened serpent power and can be observed without much difficulty by any competent investigator in whom the force is aroused.

The awakening of *kundalini* takes two distinct forms. One is the upward flow of a radiant energy that appears like a luminous glow in and around the head, and the other is the streaming of a fine biochemical essence into the brain and the nerve centers of the vital organs. The latter manifestation gives rise to distinct sensations, both in the central canal and the nerves affected by the movement.

Although the awareness of the peculiar sensations is a purely subjective experience, I am convinced that the actual movements of the organic essence should also be objectively measurable. The pleasurable sensations experienced in the play of love or the agonizing stabs of pains are also a subjective experience, but they have objective aspects that can be measured by various methods. The arousal of *kundalini* and the flow of the reproductive essences, with the component radiant psychic energy, are similarly not only simple subjective experiences, but also have definite somatic symptoms. It is for this reason that I am emphatic that the phenomenon of *kundalini* provides the much needed empirical corrobortaion of every genuine form of mystical experience.

There can be no doubt that an enhanced activity of the brain cannot be possible without the consumption of more psychic energy or alternately, without the action of a more potent form of this energy than is used by average human beings. The mysterious force behind every form of nerve activity and sensation, the hidden cause behind the electrical discharges in the nervous system and the brain, is still a riddle to science. It is in this amazing transformation of psychic energy, about which we are still in the dark, that the whole mystery of Kundalini-Yoga lies. Investigation into the phenomenon of *kundalini*, which brings into the orbit of our observation new areas of activity of the highly elusive psychic force, is perhaps the surest way at present to understand its method of work and its nature in living organisms.

It is surprising that even intelligent observers are sometimes deceived into the belief that transcendental consciousness is merely a passive and semiconscious state of mind, similar to that induced by hypnosis or that which precedes sleep, or intervenes between sleep and full waking consciousness. Since the mystical state is entirely unportrayable, one who has not had the experience can never even remotely frame a mental picture of it. Many teachers of Yoga who lack the Supreme Vision deceive themselves and those whom they instruct when they confuse passive mental states with the expanded state of consciousness called *turiya*, mentioned with reverence in the ancient treatises. It is the indescribable, marvelous state of tremendously enhanced awareness that the great mystics and seers tried, with all the force of language at their command, to delineate faithfully. But they always failed in the attempt. Modern confusion on this question is mainly due to the ignorance prevailing about the basic facts of *samadhi*, or mystical trance, not only because a picture of the condition is so difficult to convey, but also because the phenomenon has been and still is so extremely rare and unidentifiable.

From the data that I am putting into the hands of science, the verification of the mystical condition should be possible by observation of certain external symptoms that invariably follow the opening of the *brahmarandra* (the "cavity of Brahma"), leading to transhuman states of consciousness peculiar to mystics and Yoga adepts. The union of *shakti* (luminous *prana* or bioenergy and the reproductive essence) with *shiva* (the conscious principle) occurs when the stream of ambrosia enters the *brahmarandra* and floods the brain, causing an exhilaration and a rapture as if literally a fountain of intensely blissful nectar has suddenly started to pour forth its contents. Consciousness expands in radiating waves far beyond the limits of the body, then of the surrounding objects, and finally beyond the cosmic image present in the mind, until it assumes a colossal proportion beyond the range of all that can be conceived by the mind or perceived by the senses. It is this unbounded universe of consciousness, in which the enlightened Yogi, who has attained to the Sahaja state, lives perennially and has his being.

It is this transformed consciousness, elevated to cosmic proportions, that the ancient seers of India designated by the name of Brahman, Shiva, Vishnu, Nirvana, and so forth, and it is for this reason that an adept, possessing this form of transhuman awareness, is considered to be an incarnation of Shiva or Vishnu or any deity.

The very fact that mystical ecstasy gives rise to the impression that one is in communion with the Creator or has become one with Him is enough to convey the overwhelming proportions of the vision perceived. Descriptions of this state, rendered by all great seers and mystics during the past thousands of years, form the most sublime literature in the possession of mankind. With this position before the mind, the claims made that the visions of God or any other deity can be induced by hypnosis or drugs appear ridiculous in the extreme.

Let us consider the two Hindu divine incarnations, Rama and Krishna. Both are said to have been of a dusky color. In India their complexion is described as "shyam Varna," that is, of the color of the sky at dusk. According to the traditional mode of depicture, both are portrayed with form and face blue like the sky. In *turiya*, the transcendental state of consciousness, the inner illumination resembles the sky at dusk, just beginning to glow with the shimmering luster of the starry host. The body of Shiva is of an ashen hue to resemble also the silvery luster of the star-spangled sky. Some ascetics in India smear their bodies with ashes in imitation of the body of Shiva, not only as an emblem of purification, symbolizing the burning away of desire and lust, but also as a sign of Cosmic Consciousness. The saffron robes worn by others serve the same purpose, to indicate the flamelike nature of *kundalini*.

The luminosity in the head changes its hues and may resemble molten gold or the dazzling radiance of the noonday sun. "May the Goddess Tripura, who prevails in the three states of wakefulness, dreaming, and deep slumber," says the Panchastavi, "shining in the forehead like the lustrous bow of Indra [rainbow], in the crown of the head like the luminous white orb of the moon, and in the heart like the never-setting splendorous sun . . . speedily destroy all our impurities."

■ *What is the difference between the altered states of consciousness experienced with the use of drugs such as LSD, mescalin, nitrous oxide, and the like, and the genuine mystical states? In these states, according to published accounts, there definitely occurs an enhancement in the perception of colors. There are also sensations of luminosity and flashing lights. The objects observed seem to convey new meanings, and sometimes there is a sense of identification between the subject and the objects perceived. There even arises a sense of enhanced knowledge about the universe. How then do we discriminate between these drug experiences and turiya or transcendental states of consciousness?*

A critical study of various accounts of mystical experience, with a searching eye for the bodily conditions described, should leave no doubt in the minds of impartial observers that the extraordinary mental phenomena described have an unmistakable link with the state of the physical organism. With firsthand accounts like my own—and those of others who have had the experience—it should not be difficult to initiate experiments to determine and measure the biological aspects. Up until now much research has been directed to drug experiences that are entirely subjective, with, perhaps, transient changes in the chemistry of the body. These experiences do not involve any positive biological transformation, but often physical and moral degeneration.

At first sight, mystical experience and the drug state appear to have some features in common. Drugs, such as those mentioned, do produce enhancement in the perception of colors, and there are those sensations of luminosity and flashing lights and even a sense of enhanced knowledge about the universe. However, there is a world of difference between a drugtaker and a mystic. The altered states of consciousness induced by drugs evince a blunting of the intellect and a partial, if not entire, loss of the critical faculty. A sense of dizziness and unreality is almost always present, and the emotional balance is upset.

One may find a cause for boisterous laughter in a commonplace object that presents no ludicrous feature to a normal person, or there may be a sense of depression or fear associated with objects that possess no feature to evoke these emotions. The sense of deep meaning or of tremendously enhanced knowledge, even if actually present and not merely imagined, is transitory. It not only vanishes on coming back to normal consciousness but even leaves a sense of emptiness, a void where there should have been satisfaction at the attainment of new knowledge not possessed before. The subject feels in no way further elevated or transformed. On the other hand, the entry back to the normal state may be attended by lassitude, langor, a sense of nausea, accompanied by physical symptoms of a distressing nature.

Often, the novel states create an addiction to the drug and a disinclination to perform one's everyday duties. Lost in his dreams, the addict evades his responsibilities. The experience blunts his mental and moral evolution and promises a spurious "transcendentalism" without having to work for it.

Mystical experience is an altogether different proposition. The visionary or trance state is so enrapturing and fascinating that the whole being of the mystic or Yogi is irresistibly drawn toward the inner and outer display that unfolds itself before his vision. The mind becomes rapt in the contemplation of a new, glorious, inner state of consciousness, or of transformed scenes present before the outer eye. It seems as if heaven, with all its splendor and grandeur, has descended on earth to enwrap all the objects viewed, both internal and external, in a mantle of glory, beauty, and peace that is impossible to experience in the normal state. There is no blunting of the intellect, no haziness of mind, no aberrant distortion or alteration of light, color, shade, or shape. The self-recorded experiences of mystics, seers, and Yoga adepts bear ample testimony to this fact. There is no diminution of the observing power of the intellect or its measure of assessment even in the highest states of ecstasy. If it were not so, then no adept or mystic would have been able to describe his experience with such accuracy and vividness, making such life stories and narratives of superearthly experiences so appealing and fascinating for generations of human beings.

Corroboration is not far to seek. Even in this age of reason, do not the accounts left by great Christian mystics, Sufis, and the seers of India provide a fascinating and elevating study for the scholar and the layman alike? Is there any more positive evidence needed to show the great gulf existing between the lofty visions of mystics and Yoga adepts of the past and the hectic experiences caused by the ingestion of drugs? There is a world of difference between the self-revelation of the former and the accounts of the drug users of today.

The altered states of consciousness induced by drugs, hypnosis, or self-caused semitrance states of mind are all merely distorted states of normal consciousness. There may appear lights, brilliant displays of colors, sounds, flashes of creative insight, a sense of happiness and peace, and so forth, but all these varied effects are of the normal awareness, of a fevered or highly colored imagination, not of entry into a higher level of awareness of which but a small glimpse leaves one breathless with wonder and awe. It is only the tremendous potentiality present in the psychic energy released by *kundalini* that can create a change in consciousness of a magnitude that, for the duration of its operation, keeps the subject enthralled by the overwhelming and inspiring nature of the visionary experience. The accounts contained in the Agamas and Yoga manuals about the titanic state of consciousness, spread everywhere, which is introspectively apprehended by the Yogi, provide firm evidence that this is not merely an alteration of normal awareness. The perceptual faculty is not left at the same level as it was before, but a radical transformation of the observer occurs also, so that he feels one with the universe or the all-pervading or all-powerful Deity which he now perceives in his vision.

Mystical experience is not, therefore, merely an altered state of consciousness with peace, happiness, or creative intelligence, but a tremendously extended state of awareness in rapport with an unbounded sentience perceived everywhere. Peace, happiness, and creative intelligence are possessed in ample measure by common men and women who lay no claim to transcendence. Mystical experience involves a radical change in the whole area of perception, but this is not all. The genuine mystic or Yoga adept simultaneously develops extraordinary talents, psychic faculties, and creative skill. It is well known that Sufi poetry is among the richest in the whole Persian literature, and the poetry of Indian mystics and Yoga adepts like Sur Dass, Tulsi Dass, Dadu, Mira Bhai, Guru Nanak, Kabir, and others is still unequaled. It is the most popular and elevating music sung in India even today.

Scientific investigation of this extraordinary phenomenon therefore offers a vast new territory of tremendous importance. In place of so much research of a mechanistic or utilitarian nature, the subject of *kundalini* promises an inspiring work that reaches to the roots of meaning in human existence and evolution. The time is now ripe for such a renaissance.

■ *What will be the effect of the investigation into* kundalini *on modern sciences?*

The first impact of a methodical research on *kundalini* will be to open a new way of approach to the investigation of phenomena of mind and consciousness. According to current practice, psychologists depend for much of their exploration of mind on data provided by insanity, neurosis, fixations, obsessions, and other morbid states of mind, as well as dreams. But since almost nothing is known about the psychic force that is the cause of all these varied manifestations of consciousness, the investigations made so far have not been conclusive, and the whole subject is still shrouded in doubt and dispute. Other areas of psychology concerned with personality testing and aptitude are purely utilitarian, and throw no light on the rationale of mind.

Even explanations of the basic facts of insanity, genius, and mystical experience vary considerably, due to radical differences of opinion about them among psychologists of different schools of thought. The study of the effects of an awakened *kundalini* will definitely throw a flood of light on this still-obscure domain and provide a firm basis for an all-out effort to investigate the phenomena of mind. I am confident about this because the amazing knowledge of human psychology and paranormal states of consciousness, displayed by ancient Indian savants, owes its origin to the observation of the phenomenon of *kundalini*. Conducted with modern methods of study and combined with current knowledge of physiology, the investigation is certain to yield most valuable data for the understanding of consciousness in its normal, abnormal, and paranormal manifestations.

In evaluating reliable accounts of the arousing of *kundalini*, there is a wide range of literature to study, in addition to firsthand evidence. Knowledge of *kundalini* is not confined to India alone. It was known in almost all parts of the earth, including South America and Africa. There is also reliable evidence to show that knowledge of *kundalini* was current among the elite in almost all the vanished civilizations of the past. The Caduceus of Mercury, which is an emblem of *kundalini*, was known in Assyria centuries before Egypt, under the name of the "Custodian of the Tree of Life," another appellation of the Serpent Power. It is even held that the very word *"kundalini"* is derived from the Assyrian word *"kundala,"* meaning "coiled." I do not wish to enter into discussion here as to the exact place of origin of the cult of *kundalini*, but there is no doubt that it was nowhere developed and elaborated upon as thoroughly as in India. Suffice it to say that the knowledge of this psychophysiological mechanism seems to date back to prehistoric times. It formed the pivot of most of the ancient esoteric and occult systems of mental and spiritual disciplines.

I accord preference to *kundalini* over psi phenomena for leading science to an understanding of the nature of consciousness because in dealing with psi we deal with bioenergy in its paranormal manifestations. Since bioenergy or *prana* is itself impervious to the probe of the intellect and the senses, and cannot be directly observed or detected by any instruments known to science, the utmost investigators can achieve would be to verify the phenomena exhibited, such as clairvoyance, telepathy, precognition, telekinesis, materialization, and the like. But with the current methods of observation they cannot gather any information about the energy itself. It will, therefore, continue to remain a mystery even after investigation has proved that the claims are genuine. If it is conclusively demonstrated that psi phenomena do occur, but without any understanding of causation and the forces involved, this would not substantially extend the present narrow horizons of the human mind. Material objectives would continue to dominate the thinking of mankind, leading to a stultification of the evolutionary impulse and atrophy of the evolutionary mechanism, the vicious precursors of degeneration and decay.

On the other hand, research on *kundalini* implies study of the psychophysiological organism of man to determine the nature of the biological processes responsible for the generation of the psychic force at the root of all transhuman states of consciousness and paranormal faculties, including psi phenomena. Almost all enlightened seers in India, including Buddha, are in agreement over the fact that healthy forms of Yoga and spiritual disciplines lead to the development of psychic faculties, and that the practitioners should abstain from making use of them to avoid distraction on the path of self-unfoldment. Since *kundalini* is the biological lever responsible for success in every form of spiritual exercise, it naturally follows that the same lever is also responsible for the development of psi faculties, which form a corollary to spiritual awakening. We are surely right, therefore, in holding that *kundalini* should be the prime objective of research.

Scientists should note that cases of awakening of *kundalini* are not as uncommon as is usually supposed. But since knowledge about this mechanism is extremely restricted, and the masses continue to be in ignorance about it, those individuals who have a spontaneous awakening at one time or another often fail to recognize their own symptoms and attribute the extraordinary states that they experience to some freakish display of the mind or to abnormality. I receive many letters from people, both in the East and the West, who gain new insights into their own experience upon reading the accounts in my book* or in some other works on the subject and wish to be more fully enlightened about their condition and to know more facts about the power. If this has happened with the circulation of only a few thousand copies of a few books, what will be the position when knowledge about *kundalini* becomes widespread in different countries and among all classes of people? It will then be found, as I believe should be the case at the present level of evolution, that hundreds of thousands of people all over the world—especially among intellectuals—do have experiences of *kundalini* in one form or another.

■ Let us suppose that someone has a spontaneous experience of kundalini and has no knowledge about its nature or working. Wouldn't it be risky for such a person to be without guidance and have to depend on his own resources for dealing with the situation?

Certainly there are countless cases of spontaneous awakening of *kundalini* of which no cognizance is taken at any stage. Unfortunately, some of these trail off into insanity, because the

---

* *Kundalini, the Evolutionary Energy in Man.*

experience is not understood and proper advice is not available. It is an irony of fate that at this critical juncture in the evolutionary development of mankind the world should be in deplorable ignorance about this vital mechanism, known under different names not only in India, but in Egypt, Mesopotamia, China, South America, and Greece many centuries ago. The investigation into the causes leading to psychosis must ultimately lead to the same conclusions that I am here presenting, namely, that in a certain percentage of cases the malady is due to a morbid functioning of the evolutionary mechanism brought about by various causes.

Apart from psychosis, there are also many people in whom the awakening of *kundalini* leads to neurosis and other psychic disorders. They lead an unbalanced life without crossing the border into the territory of the incurably insane. There are also others who, while having the experiences, manage to continue in the normal tenor of their lives. By study or contact with others who possess knowledge on the subject, they come to understand something of the cause responsible for their extraordinary experiences. An investigation into a number of such cases is sure to bring to light valuable scientific facts about *kundalini*.

The current methods of treatment often do not succeed in such cases, because nothing is yet known about the evolutionary mechanism in human beings. I remember very well the case of a friend who experienced a definite symptom of *kundalini* awakening and went with his story to a psychologist. The latter said that such a phenomenon was quite unknown in the domain of psychology and that it must be a delusion of some sort or an unconscious impulse finding its way into surface consciousness. I am sure that if a committee of dedicated scientists set up a research project on *kundalini*, they will find no difficulty in locating numerous such cases.

Empirical verification of *kundalini* is most likely to lead to an

explosion in the thinking of mankind, because it has no precedent in history. Because of the tremendous possibilities involved,
having a most direct bearing on the life of each individual, the
upheaval caused will far exceed the effect of the Copernican
revolution and every other great discovery of science made during recent times. Guided by instincts, mankind carried on for
thousands of years without the knowledge that the earth re-
volved around the sun, or that the stars and planets were held in
space by the force of gravity, or that the surface of the moon has
such and such a formation. Man thrived and prospered during
this vast span of time without ever coming up against such a
crisis as he is facing now, due to the prevailing ignorance about
the evolutionary mechanism. If this lack is not supplied soon, he
may suffer a disaster of unimaginable magnitude to learn the
nature of the inviolable spiritual laws that rule his destiny.

Even today, among those practising Yoga in the ashrams and
monastic institutions in India, there occur cases of *kundalini*
awakening during the course of training. Ascetics of this category are not easily accessible for investigation, but individuals
might be forthcoming who would allow observation and study
of their conditions in the interest of knowledge. With the foundation of a research organization on scientific lines, and with
wide publicity, there should be no dearth of genuine cases available for investigation. I am convinced that the data collected
even in a few instances would provide enough material for the
world of science to place *kundalini* in the category of recognized
phenomena of the human organism, needing further study and
investigation to ascertain the nature and full details of its various
spheres of manifestation. What is of importance is that the basic
facts should be ascertained and studied without preconceptions.

The following passage from *The Secret of the Golden Flower*,
a Chinese book of life, can leave no doubt that the author in-
tends to convey the inward and upward flow of the reproductive

energy, the ultimate aim of all forms of Yoga and other religious disciplines:

"The power of the kidneys is under the water sign. When the instincts are stirred, it runs downward, is directed outward and creates children. If, in the moment of release, it is not allowed to flow outward, but is led back by the force of thought, so that it penetrates the crucible of the creative, and refreshes heart and body and nourishes them, that also is the backward flowing method. Therefore it is said: 'The meaning of The Elixir of Life depends on the backward flowing method!' "

The backward flowing is the Urdhava-Retas of Indian Masters. Yet Professor Jung, in his lengthy introduction to the above book, completely missed the point and made futile attempts to incorporate this teaching within the framework of his own idolized "unconscious." In the note on page 131 he writes: "To a certain extent our text leaves open the question as to whether, by 'a continuation of life,' a survival after death or a prolongation of physical existence, is meant. Expressions such as life-elixir and the like, are insidiously obscure." It is obvious that this great psychologist had no inkling of what has been the most remarkable phenomenon in the history of civilization, namely, the transmutation of reproductive energy, leading to the two most productive states of the human mind—creativity and mystical experience. It is important, therefore, that the phenomenon of *kundalini* should be investigated without preconceptions or a desire to validate existing theories.

There are some people who continue to believe that the subtle effects of *kundalini* may be traced by standard techniques of electroencephalography. But such methods cannot measure the quality of perception. I believe that new techniques and electronic apparatus will be evolved when the phenomenon has been properly evaluated.

What is primarily needed is a receptive frame of mind, accepting the fact of the possibility of the phenomenon, based on the testimony of many outstanding intellects of the past. What is actually happening at present, however, is that even those interested in this investigation direct their efforts to the verification of the physical aspects of Yoga and not to its psychological effect, with far-reaching organic changes in the body that are characteristic of a higher state of consciousness. The study needs imaginative pioneers like Sir Jagadis Chandra Bose, whose brilliant experiments in plant reaction were made possible by his own genius in devising delicate instruments to measure the phenomenon, and who, like other present-day savants, has perfected techniques for detecting the subtle reactions of bioenergy in healthy and diseased animals and plants, without yet having gained acceptance for their results from the orthodox ranks of science.

Why research on *kundalini* is of utmost importance for mankind at this stage of its evolution is because it can directly lead to the awareness of the fact that Revelation, to which paramount importance was attached throughout the past, is as essential for the welfare and the progress of the race as genius and intellectual talent and that the Serpent Power is the organic source behind them all. Contrary to common belief, the real object of Yoga and the transcendental states of consciousness to which it leads is not merely to experience a state of bliss or to perform miraculous feats but, what is of the highest importance, to open new channels of perception by which Revelation and *jnana* (perennial wisdom) become possible. If the question is asked, What has been the greatest contribution of the founders of all major faiths and the greatest seers and sages of the past? the immediate answer would be: the revealed literature of mankind. In this priceless contribution miracles, paranormal phenomena, and the like hold no position at all!

Through all the course of history, no spiritual man ever born was able, even partially, to duplicate the miracles performed by science. The miracles of speed, of distant vision, of instant communication over enormous distances, of flying through the air or diving under the ocean, the miracles of surgery and healing, and numerous other amazing technologies cannot but inspire mankind with a confidence in the importance of logic and intellect.

■ *You refer to achievements of science, but hasn't science become destructive? Aren't the nuclear arsenals of the superpowers now a deadly threat to the very existence of the race, and dosen't the use or rather abuse of technology result in pollution of the atmosphere and the contamination of water, endangering human life everywhere?*

Knowledge can be both constructive and destructive. The ultimate arbiter is the human intellect. It is not science that has become destructive, but it is the distortion and vitiation of the human intellect that is responsible for the present unsafe situation of the world. The reason why Revelation is a necessary instrument for the spiritual progress of the race is because intellect, unable to foresee centuries or even decades ahead, cannot determine the evolutionary needs of mankind at a particular time, and is liable to make serious errors in calculation. Human life, both of the individual and society, is so complex and the course of evolution so full of bewildering situations that only a cosmic intelligence can guide it rightly to the destined goal.

Can even the highest intellects in every branch of knowledge, assisted by computers, make an accurate forecast of what will be the state of mankind after the span of only the next half century? Or can they predict the changes in the current concepts of science, politics, and religion in this period? Does this not plainly signify that the race as a whole is drifting toward an indeterminate goal at the mercy of forces over which it has no control?

The error of science has been that it has largely ignored the spiritual side of man and devoted its attention to the physical and organic fields. The outcome is that mankind faces a threat of annihilation through war, of death by poisoned air, water, and earth, and of mental and intellectual distortion because of a highly mechanical and unnatural way of life. On the political side, life has become a seething caldron of aggression, violence, hate, and lust for power. On the spiritual and moral side we see confusion rampant, for there are as many ideas, concepts, systems, and doctrines as there are teachers expounding them. It is not surprising, therefore, that science has failed to create that homogeneity and clarity of thought that is essential for the harmonious progress of mankind.

Science in our day is suffering from the same distemper of mind that affected faith during the period of the supremacy of religion, namely, dogmatism and vanity. It is amazing to what extent materialistic scientists can be led astray by vanity in separating science from spiritual understanding. They understand very well that all we know about the visible cosmos is but a drop in the ocean of knowledge, and that each year they are forced to revise their opinions about certain issues or to add more facts to the existing information. But with all this uncertainty, most of them display a dogmatic attitude toward mind and consciousness. Because science has been one-sided in this investigation, ignoring the spiritual side of man, it has failed to bring about that wholesome transformation in the mental and moral spheres as it has done on the physical plane.

The neglect of the material side in former times brought about the fall of the once highly honored sovereign faiths of mankind. Now, in a similar way, the neglect of the spiritual side is undermining the ascendency gained by science. In both cases, it was the intellect that failed to assess the position correctly and erred in overemphasizing only one side of man and neglecting the other equally important side. It is not science itself, therefore, that is at fault, but the overweening vanity and shortsightedness of overconfident savants who refuse to admit that what they know is infinitely small as compared to what they do not know.

■ *What are your suggestions, then, for a harmonious development of human beings and the eradication of present-day irrational beliefs and practices in the spiritual realm?*

The first thing I would suggest is an investigation into consciousness. We have a huge volume of literature available in India, describing methods for attaining the higher states of consciousness and the nature of these higher states. A documentary research into these volumes, followed by systematic experimentation, can, I am sure, lead to an understanding of the biological relationship between expanded mental states and the brain. When this is achieved, the next step would be to find the laws underlying this relationship. Enough material would be available in the hands of scholars and scientists then to determine the path and the goal of evolution, and to adjust human life accordingly.

One important feature of this investigation will be that with the experience gained by the observation of a few cases, more potent methods for effecting the arousal of the power and more effective measures for averting risks can be devised. Then more and more fruitful experiments can be made until sufficient data about the phenomenon is collected. These, in turn, would lead to a universal acceptance of the evolutionary mechanism and the target in front of it, resulting in the formulations of a regular science dealing with the whole subject.

All that I have to say about this amazing human potentiality constitutes but a drop in the ocean of knowledge that will emerge as soon as dedicated persons begin to devote their whole-hearted attention to it.

It can be readily imagined that this consummation cannot be achieved immediately or even in the course of a few decades, but there is no doubt that enough data would soon be collected to enable scholars to understand the nature of the changes occurring imperceptibly in the brain and consciousness. It is not only by the study of and experimentation on the methods leading to higher states of consciousness, but also by the observation of the psychic forces responsible for genius, mediumistic faculties, and insanity that these evolutionary processes can be understood and the nature of the mechanism determined.

As I have pointed out in my earlier writings, the all-inclusive nature of sex energy has not yet been correctly understood even by the leading authorities on the subject. In fact, the very term reproductive or sex energy is a misnomer; reproduction is but one of the aspects of the life-energy, of which the other theater of activity is the brain. The cephalic activity is so slow and subtle as to be almost imperceptible. It is this activity that is the cause of genius, uncanny psychic powers, and also insanity. Once this fact is empirically demonstrated, we come to a turning point in our present concepts about mind and consciousness—even about matter and the universe as a whole.

The first harvest of this change will be the beginning of a new science, dealing with subtle intelligent energies in the cosmos. When this happens the gigantic physical world—now dominating the whole mental horizon of science—will be relegated to its proper position as the visible peak of an infinite creation of which the unbounded major part is sunk below the surface of the space-time ocean, hidden from the sight of men. It is only in higher states of consciousness that a fragment of the submerged portion comes into view, causing a state of wonder and exhilaration beyond description. It is only when the evolving human organism and the cosmos upon which it depends for its existence are viewed in the right perspective, in relation to the ultimate state of consciousness designed for mankind, that the appropriate ways of life and conduct and a salubrious environment favorable to this inner transformation can be devised by science.

Try as we may, without a clear knowledge of the goal ahead we can by no exercise of the intellect determine the right pattern of life, or the right kind of milieu, essential for mankind on the evolutionary path.

A united world, abolition of war, demolition of armaments, disbandment of armies, an environment more in harmony with nature, a life more natural and simple, removal of barriers between man and man, inculcation of altruistic and humanitarian principles, moral education, social equality, and universal brotherhood are some of the basic factors contributing to the harmonious progress of mankind.

What I say may appear idealistic or even fantastic and impracticable to many people. But for one in rapport with the cosmic plane of consciousness, the conclusion is unavoidable. At its present intellectual stature, the alternatives facing the race are either self-caused annihilation, with dreadful agony for myriads, or knowledge of and obedience to the laws of evolving consciousness.

It is amazing how shortsighted we mortals can be. The whole mighty scheme of evolution is designed to carry mankind toward a sublime state of consciousness and a lofty mode of life. It means to usher in an era of such happiness, peace, and plenty, and a life of such fulfillment and bliss, that we cannot frame even a distant picture of it in our wildest dreams. Denied the glorious vision of this cosmic plane, and tied to the earth with unbreakable chains of ambition and desire, even the most far-sighted thinkers, building their picture of the future on conditions existing at present, fail to appreciate that but a single turn of events can create such a global upheaval in human thought, or cause such a purgatorial revolution, that a purified humanity may emerge to act, with all the resources at its command, to build a war-free, glorious world to abide in.

We need not turn to history for a confirmation of these views. There is no precedent in the past of such devastating forces at the command of man, such preparedness for mutual destruction, and such a slender margin between the safety of the race and its total death as is the position at present. Mankind is face to face with such a situation for the first time, and the experience gained now, pleasant or bitter, will provide an historical precedent for the future of life itself.

■ *If the existence of an evolutionary goal is empirically demonstrated, how can this help to clear the present confusion? So many educated people still continue to express divergent views, even concerning the empirically demonstrated truths of science.*

There will, of course, continue to exist some conflicts of opinions even when the truths of what I assert are experimentally proved. But such conflict will relate to the details, the causes at the base, the relative potency of the various methods and the like, not to the fundamental facts of the mechanism and the evolutionary target.

To illustrate, let us take the law of gravity, the theory of relativity, or the doctrine of evolution. Although there are still differences of view about some of the yet unresolved issues, there is a general agreement about the broad principles involved. For instance, with the doctrine of evolution, it is now generally admitted that the only way to account for the appearance of life on earth is to assume a process of evolution from the simplest forms slowly developing into more complex ones. Whether this process of development resulted from chance, mutation, or from inherent tendencies striving toward a predetermined pattern, has yet to be ascertained.

In the same way, when we once accept that in the case of man, biological evolution toward a higher state of consciousness provides the springhead for all the phenomena connected with religion, this will lend a different color to the whole realm of the divine and the supernatural. It would then be clearly realized that it is not to propitiate a god or any other spiritual entity that one has to pay attention to the dictums of faith; but that the principle of evolutionary progress toward a spiritual goal has to be accepted in a way similar to the principle of growth and development of a child toward sane and healthy maturity.

Although there is no unanimity of opinion about the best way to bring up a child, the process of growth is universally recognized. Every parent has his own views about it, and we see this diversity also reflected in the accepted educational systems in various countries. However, this diversity and conflict of view does not detract from the patent fact that the child has to grow to manhood, and that all the intelligence and all the resources of the parents should be directed to make this process of growth happy, safe, and most fruitful.

One immediate result of the demonstration of the evolutionary goal will be that a good deal of public attention will be diverted from negative activities toward the clarification of this colossal issue. Scholars and laity alike will voice their opinions, and the press will resound with discussions. The pens of writers

and journalists will be busy presenting the case both for and
against the new concept, subjecting every article, dogma, and
doctrine to ruthless analysis, leading ultimately to a thorough
overhauling of the whole unwieldly structure of religion.

Another salutary effect of this ferment and upheaval would be
that the false founders of spurious cults, the imposters, racke-
teers—all those misguided men and women who, in order to exploit to advantage the burning spiritual thirst in human hearts
and make this sacred province an arena for the satisfaction of their
own desire for power, wealth, name, or fame—will gradually disappear from the scene. When it is firmly established that the
ultimate reward of Yoga or other religious disciplines is the
crown of Cosmic Consciousness—of oneness with the beatific,
deathless ocean of existence—then who would like to barter away
the diadem of life eternal for fragile trinkets of earthly success or
phychic gifts?

Can there be a greater miracle than creation or than life itself?
Those in whom the contemplation of the star-spangled sky on a
clear night, or the spectacle of the rolling ocean, or a vast panorama of nature can evoke feelings of wonder, awe, and adoration
in regard to the Almighty Author of this marvelous whole are
not likely to be impressed by the displays of those who resort to
thaumaturgy, sleight-of-hand, or enchantment to mystify the
uninformed and create a belief in their own superhuman stature
and powers.

Transition from the present-day concepts of religion and the
occult toward the philosophy of evolution involves so radical a
change in thinking that even the most imaginative men may not
be able to envisage the consequences. Once the evolutionary interpretation is admitted, it will clarify and transform the exposi-
tions of great teachers of spirituality and religion, past and present. The energy generated in millions of people by the insatiable
hunger for supernatural experiences will not be frittered away

then in improvising, maintaining, and spreading hundreds of novel, mysterious, sectarian, or obscure creeds and cults. Rather, it will go toward inculcating true knowledge about the evolutionary target prescribed for man and devising healthy universal methods for its attainment.

Throughout the past, there have been scores of mass movements, as at present, but the noise dwindled down, after the death of the founders, with the realization of contradictions and falsities in their creeds. The same will befall the hollow mass movements of our day, religious or political. Truth persists, even though it may appear only in tiny proportions in the beginning. It gathers mass like an avalanche, sweeping away everything that obstructs its path. I am certain that the concept of *kundalini* in evolution will gain acceptance.

It is not my desire that the concept be accepted unquestioningly and that people try to awaken *kundalini* in the belief it will provide a panacea for all the ills of the world. On the contrary, it will be my first endeavor to arrange an investigation of the phenomenon under the supervision of competent observers, men of both faith and science. Even when the experiments are successful and the principle demonstrated, there will be no attempt to enlist disciples and followers or to found a new sect or cult. Every effort will be directed to educating the public about the divine power always mysteriously at work in their systems, both in wakefulness and sleep, to make them aware of their responsibility to lead a life in consonance with the demands of this mighty, irresistible force.

The growth of knowledge is resistless. During the last two centuries almost the entire attention of science was directed toward the investigation of physical phenomena and the discovery of the laws and properties of matter. If we now look retrospectively at the convulsions and spasms that attended the birth of modern science, because of the often hostile attitude of faith, we will not feel surprised at the cold and negative attitude shown by so many great savants toward the problems of religion, or to be more precise, toward the phenomenon of life and consciousness. It is as if some hidden tendency of the mind barred the way to it. The entry of modern psychology into the ranks of regular science first broke the ice of this chilly attitude. Now we are witnessing the very reverse of what was observed during the course of development of materialistic science. The riddle of consciousness now looms large before the mental horizon of not only the masses but the intellectuals as well.

Those who through erroneous preconceptions now show a skeptical or lukewarm attitude toward those ideas are sure to witness the swing of the pendulum. Everything about the disclosures I am making I have experienced myself. I have confirmed my experience with the traditional concepts relating to this esoteric science that have been known and verified during the past thousands of years. Hence I am as sure of the authenticity of what I state and of the ultimate acceptance of this truth as I am of the fact that summer is invariably followed by autumn and winter by spring.

7   *Kundalini* in the Evolution of Mankind

■ *How would kundalini effect the present social and political structure of mankind?*

The present social structure of mankind is built on the assumption that the human brain has reached its peak and that every individual is expected to derive the maximum benefit and happiness by the best exercise of his strength, skill, or talent for as long a period as he can possibly do so. There is generally no appreciation of the important fact that in order not to interfere with or obstruct the processes of evolution ceaselessly active in the body it is absolutely necessary that the mode of life should be concordant to the mighty impulse and that a proper balance be maintained between periods of rest and exertion of the body and brain.

Other forms of life maintain this balance instinctively, but man has to discover it for himself. The observation of the rhythm is all the more necessary for him because of the more complex structure of his brain and the unavoidable demands of the evolutionary processes molding it into an even more complex pattern than before. This being so, each individual has to ascertain, by watching the reactions of his organism, what amount of rest and exertion is best suited to his constitution. At first sight, such meticulous observation of oneself may appear too cumbersome to some people to be made a regular feature of life. This is a great error and has already done much damage to mankind. A moment's reflection is enough to show the logical necessity of such observation.

Since self-willed man is now an active partner in the evolutionary activity of his organism, it is evident that in order to allow the activity to continue unimpeded, he must learn to shape his own mode of life and behavior to assist the evolutionary drive. The revealed scriptures of all major faiths can leave no doubt that, from the very beginning, the object of Revelation has been to prescribe practical rules of conduct and ways of life with the avowed object of salvation or self-unfoldment. There is no system or religious discipline that does not lay particular emphasis on a certain mode of conduct and behavior as a prerequisite for gaining success in the undertaking.

Studied with care, the revealed scriptures of mankind will be found to be economical directions for the regulation of human life, interspersed with myths, allegories, prophetic utterances, divine exhortations, promises of reward, and threats of punishment in this life and the next. They are regarded as inspired documents, purporting to reveal the path by which man can attain to his Maker, or gain liberation from the ever-rotating wheel of life and death. If we now substitute the concept of a more advanced state of consciousness, partaking of the divine, in place of the concepts of Brahman, Tao, Ishwara, Jehovah, Allah, Nirvana, or God, the whole volume of revealed commandments, whatever the faith to which they relate, could very well serve the purpose of rational ordinances for the regulation of human life to meet the demands of evolution.

Ideas of identification with a supreme deity arise because man has come to regard himself as only next in rank to the Creator. In such a state of mind, the obvious meaning he could place upon the glimpses of the higher state of existence of a few re-

ligious geniuses could only be that these personages had won to
the presence of the Lord God Himself.

Thousands of divines, scholars, and metaphysicians, who ex-
patiated or commented on such experiences, almost invariably
attributed them to Divine favor, in other words, to the working
of the Divine Will demanding that man should seek his Creator
and in the intensity of love absorb himself into Him. According
to the Indian tradition, it is only after millions of births (eight
million, four hundred thousand, to be exact) that the ascend-
ing soul attains the form of a human being and thereafter, striving incessantly, again through innumerable births, eventually
can win to a stature where union with Ishwara or Brahman becomes possible. For the Buddhists, Nirvana is the ultimate
heaven for the incessantly transmigrating elements of the soul.
For the followers of Semitic religions, attainment of God or
Allah is the ultimate aim of a righteous life. In short, the aim of
every religious doctrine has been to treat the human consciousness as the summit of life beyond which only God reigned in His
glory.

The main factor responsible for such a parochial view has been
the arrogance of man, bolstered by his isolation from other varieties of life in the universe. This arrogance has not been confined only to faith but has also invaded the realm of science. The
tremendous advances in our concepts of the universe, resulting
from improved methods of study and observation, should have
led to a reorientation in thinking about our insignificant position
in creation, but instead it has tended to add to our conceit by
assigning a unique position to man as the only rational being in
a cosmos of billions of luminous worlds. It is not surprising then
that a paradoxical situation still continues to exist. On the one
hand, the believers continue to insist that man is built in the
image of God or is latently God (Brahman) Himself, and the
sole object of his life is to gain communion with his Maker.

While on the other hand, the unbelievers, eliminating God altogether from creation, usurp His place and assign to man the position of supremacy in a boundless stretch of lifeless worlds of fire, floating aimlessly in space, without conveying a single hint about the purpose of their aeonic existence.

In holding to such assumptions, no room seems to have been left for the idea that the human brain can attain to other dimensions of consciousness in which the universe presents a completely different picture. In fact, because of our utter ignorance concerning the evolutionary mechanism and its laws, we are constantly impeding or arresting the evolutionary processes, although also furthering or accelerating them unconsciously by our efforts in the right directions. But the superintelligent *prana* or vital energy modifies the effect of our derelictions and digressions to an extent that makes it possible to keep the human brain in a constant state of slow progress toward its evolutionary goal. It is only when the derelictions and digressions exceed a certain limit that a process of deterioration and degeneration begins.

I can safely assert that the progress made by mankind in any direction, from the subhuman level to the present, has been far less due to man's own efforts than to the activity of the evolutionary forces at work within him. Every incentive to invention, discovery, aesthetics, and the development of improved social and political organizations invariably comes from within, from the depths of his consciousness by the grace of *kundalini*—the superintelligent Evolutionary Force in human beings.

■ *If what you say is admitted as true, it means that* kundalini *commands a large sphere of influence in the mental constitution of human beings, and we may have to accept it as a most vital part of human life such as the brain, the heart, lungs,*

*stomach, and other important organs in the body on which our
existence depends.*

You are perfectly right. I should say that the psychophysiological mechanism of *kundalini* is as important for the existence,
health, and happiness of human beings as any of their vital
organs, and as necessary for the continuance and survival of the
race as the reproductive system, perhaps even more, for the reason that the generation of the very current of life of humanity
depends on the healthy functioning of the evolutionary powerhouse.

We all know the tremendous influence exerted by the reproductive urge on the life of every man and woman. Some modern
psychologists have gone so far as to ascribe the growth of civilization and culture and even the development of talents in gifted
individuals directly or indirectly to the expressions of the sexual
force. Freud will be remembered mainly for his challenging
views about the important role played by the reproductive urge
in all spheres of human activity and thought. According to
Freudian psychology, repressed sexual desire is one of the chief
causative factors in insanity and neurosis.

There is no sphere of human activity, including even religion,
that is immune from the depredations of the sexual urge. The
whole literary and dramatic output of mankind revolves directly
or indirectly around the relationship between men and women.
The world of entertainment is built around the same fundamental theme. Even our dreams are a hunting ground for this
most compulsive impulse. Is there any other factor that has a
more powerful effect on our thoughts, fancies, and dreams, from
the age of puberty to the end of life, than sex? It is obvious that
nature has planted this urge so deeply in the whole fabric of our
being that escape from, or negation of, it is difficult or even impossible. Those who attempt this formidable task have often

had to pay a heavy cost for its suppression in one way or another.

The evolutionary impulse is no less strong and no less marked, with all the features that characterize the reproductive urge. The main difference lies in the fact that on account of the extremely slow speed of evolutionary processes, and their imperceptible nature, the effects caused are not immediately obvious and lack the violent and powerful reactions of an excited or repressed sexual impulse. But although tardy in effect, a repressed, thwarted, or violated evolutionary impulse can be even more disastrous than repressed sex, not only to individuals but also to groups and nations—even to the whole of mankind.

Let us consider the causes underlying the bloody revolutions of recent history. The main reason responsible for the upheaval and the violence in most cases was the tyranny of an oppressive political order that provoked the hatred of the people subjected to it. But we also find that the very same systems had been in existence for centuries without creating such hatred or such violent reactions from the multitudes, who had more or less formerly submitted tamely to them.

We can cite numerous parallels in history where people in different lands yielded submissively to exactions, extortions, oppression, and even barbarity of their kings, feudal lords, or emperors for centuries without once raising their heads in revolt. Then all of a sudden at a certain point of saturation a rebellion broke out. The point is, why should a multitude that, at one time, had dumbly submitted to exploitation and tyranny, without question, at another time, even under more benign conditions, resort to revolt and bloodshed to overthrow the hated regime?

The answer to this question is hard to find unless we accept that there is an evolutionary impulse at work in the race, both in individuals and the mass. This impulse finds expression through specially constituted individuals, whom we classify as "revolutionaries," who create an upheaval to overthrow an obsolete system that acts as a serious obstacle to the evolutionary drive.

The same is true of some of the ancient cultures, such as those of Greece and Rome. In their case also revolutionary political and religious ideas took possession of the minds of the people at the instigation of unconforming intellectuals at a certain point of mental development. A similar reformation of social, political, and religious institutions occurred in India in the heyday of the Vedic culture. The same phenomenon was repeated when the European mind attained to new levels of thought after the Renaissance.

It is obvious, therefore, that it is not only the spread of education or instigation by fiery revolutionaries that leads to political upheavals, but there must also have become manifest a certain degree of preparedness in the mental soil of the multitudes that enabled the seed of revolt to grow and spread until it permeated the whole mass. The constant improvement in political orders and systems of administration witnessed from the dawn of history, subject of course to vicissitudes and regressions, represents a clearly recognizable phenomenon of evolution. The political orders underwent changes in order to become more democratic and egalitarian in consonance with the evolutionary demand of the human mind.

The moment we accept that the human brain is in a state of growth to attain a predetermined wider state of cognition, we must also concede that this evolution can only be possible if the social, political, and religious orders of a people or the whole of mankind keep pace with this development.

Most of us would, no doubt, shrink at the mere idea of a modern intellectual delighting in a religious sacrifice or orgy such as characterized prehistoric times, and would unhesitatingly label such an individual as a lunatic or pervert. Similarly the very idea of living under a medieval system of government, in which whole populations considered themselves, their families, and all they owned as the chattels of a lord, liege, or prince, would appear obnoxious to a modern mind.

There was a time when a slave was a legitimate possession of his master and slavery an unquestionable accepted social institution. There was no direct condemnation of slavery even from a humanitarian like Christ, although the evil was rampant in His day. For centuries hardly any voice was raised against the loathsome institution of untouchability in India. It continued to thrive and flourish for epochs before the mind of man grasped the injustice and inhumanity involved. Torture, another inhuman institution, was accepted until relatively recent times as a legitimate instrument of law, until evolving human intellect realized the atrocity and the brutality involved in it. The modern trends to abolish war and capital punishment or to improve conditions in lunatic asylums and jails are humane movements of the same category, designed to place social and political systems on a level commensurate with the evolutionary stature of the race.

The state of perennial flux in the social, political, and religious systems of mankind is due to the activity of the evolutionary force in human beings. We know very well that no other form of life from the fish to the anthropoids possesses the mental flexibility to come out of the instinctual rut that regulates its social behavior. Man alone has this capacity because he is still in a state of transition toward a higher dimension of life. There is also evidence that when the evolutionary mechanism becomes atrophied through unfavorable climatic conditions, complete isolation, or inimical social and religious customs—as in the case of some segregated primitive populations—a people may not advance even a step beyond the boundary reached by their distant palaeolithic ancestors more than fifteen to twenty thousand years ago.

Old orders change to yield place to new ones because in order to survive, every order must conform to the rising evolutionary level of the race. The establishment of more liberal forms of government and more equitable laws did not originate merely from the greater knowledge and experience gained by mankind during the course of its thousands of years of cultural existence, but because of the growing humanistic tendencies in the mind. If this were not so, no amount of intelligence or education could keep the human mind from developing sadistic and inhuman traits.

In all cases of ethical development, it is not merely reason but psychic factors and evolutionary causes that are mainly responsible for them. For instance, the bombing and massacre of civilians—innocent men, women, and children—that has been a common feature of wars fought during this century, and the employment of that atrocious engine of destruction, the nuclear bomb, provides an anachronism that must eventually be discarded. Another evolutionary step is needed to arouse the modern conscience to the sheer brutality of waging war on unarmed and defenseless civilians, and the insanity of using atomic weapons that can cause the destruction of the whole race. When this arousal of conscience will crystallize we have yet to see, but it can be confidently asserted that after perhaps a few decades our own progeny will condemn us for this brutal disposition, as we now condemn the authors of historical massacres of the past.

I must stress, with all the emphasis at my command, that every step in the inner purification of our minds from the savage to the present stage has occurred through the evolutionary processes at work in the human body. It is only the activity of *kundalini* that keeps the evolving human mind sane and sound. Night and day we transgress the still inscrutable laws of life, abuse our organs and in a hundred ways, both in thought and deed, act in a manner prejudicial to the reformative processes active within ourselves. It is only the favor of this divine force that, acting without our awareness, heals the injured cells and revitalizes the weak areas in our brains to enable the evolutionary adjustments to proceed unimpeded.

We are not at all aware of this uninterrupted activity in our bodies, shut out as we are from the finer strata of creation, too subtle to be perceived by our senses. We fail to observe the movements of intelligent superphysical forces that course through our bodies, stimulating or restraining the billions of neurons in our brain and the unceasing activity of the nervous system. Our changing moods are the result of endless variations in the composition of the psychic elements that form the background for our personality. An insane or neurotic mind lacks the ability to reason itself into the assurance that the hallucinations it sees or the moods of depression and excitement that it experiences are but the creations of its own imagination and have no validity for others.

The least impurity or disorientation of *prana*, the vital energy that forms the basis of our personality and determines the pattern of our mind and intellect, leads to perverse and disordered thinking without the subject being aware of the fault in his behavior or mode of thought. We have little or no control over the inherent tendencies of our mind and often fall prey to misconceptions and delusions without awareness of the defect.

Whole nations, dynasties, families as well as individuals can fall prey to degenerative, perverse, or insane tendencies without awareness of the downward or abnormal trends, continuing to believe that they are thinking and behaving in the right manner, justifying their departures from the prescribed or normal mode with pseudologic twisted to suit the warped frame of their minds. In this way, millions who take to drugs and errant ways of life become rebels to society and its existing fabric under the delusion that they are acting and behaving in the right way. If it were not for the processes of inner purification and adjustment, the whole pattern of human thinking could change into abnormal or distorted expressions resistlessly, without awareness of the shift.

The best measures to be employed for the continued evolutionary progress of the race should not only be effective in counteracting the degenerative tendencies, but also in maintaining the activity of the evolutionary processes at the proper pitch at all times. This is a more difficult proposal than may appear at first sight, because each human being is such a complex bundle of emotions, passions, desires, and ambitions, and has such a varied range of patterns of feeling, thinking, and acting, that it is not possible to prescribe a standard method uniformly effective for all people for all time to come. At every fresh step on the scale of evolution, new methods have to be devised and prescribed, for which Revelation will invariably come to guide the human race.

The most important step needed to be taken at present is to educate the rank and file about the evolutionary activity of every human organism. After this knowledge is widely disseminated, healthy and safe methods for accelerating the processes can be prescribed. The methods can be selected after a careful examination and trial from the host of practices, exercises, and disciplines described in all the esoteric and occult doctrines, religious documents, and Yoga manuals at present extant. They can be weighed and tested in the scale of the scientific knowledge of today. This will need laborious research on the part of a team of dedicated workers for a number of years.

When the task is completed, the methods and the practices chosen can be made a part of the educational systems at present in use, and applied in graduated steps adapted to different constitutions and to different stages of life. Once this is done, the whole spiritual education and discipline of mankind will become a regular science, the most important part of human knowledge.

When this comes to pass, weird cults and sects will gradually cease to exist; the cobwebs of dogma and doubt surrounding every major religious creed will be swept away, and spiritual discipline become a part of human life, as general education for the mind and hygiene of the body are today.

It is unfortunate that there is as yet no adequate modern equivalent to the ancient Hindu science of *kundalini*, for the terminology, rooted in the religious concepts of its day, becomes associated with the modern miracle-mongers of East and West, and cults of instant "enlightenment" or "transcendentalism." This creates much confusion, and modern scientists often become prejudiced at what appears to them to be outdated religion or modern charlatanism. It is to be hoped that the researches I am recommending will result in a terminology and conceptual system acceptable to modern science. Meanwhile, however, the basic framework and terminology of the science of *kundalini*, so superbly developed by ancient seers, must stand as the only reliable guide to a system of knowledge unknown to modern scientists.

Kundalini has as varied an expression in all spheres of human activity—spiritual, moral, intellectual, physical, academic, therapeutic, sexual, aesthetic, and the rest—as life itself. I am confident that the very first cases of awakened *kundalini* will bring momentous facts to the attention of the scientists engaged on this research. This will mark the beginning of the glorious career ordained for mankind. With the appropriate development of the moral, physical, and mental sides of man, new and unexpected horizons of progress will open for the race. Only a fraction of the whole unbounded kingdom of mind is at present accessible to scholars. Even the huge volume of literature that has grown up during the last century since psychology found admission to the rank of sciences is still a nebulous mass of speculations so far as the basic issues are concerned. The nature and action of the *prana* (bioenergy) that feeds the brain and the nervous system has yet to be precisely determined.

It is not difficult to imagine what profound changes will emerge in the thinking of scientists when it is definitely proved that the whole gamut of evolution, from primordial life-forms to the bewildering complexity of the organic kingdom, has occurred mainly through changes in the spectrum of bioenergy. This intelligent cosmic medium is as responsible for the phenomenon of embodied life as material energy for the emergence of the physical world. The living electricity that is the cause of animation of every cell and every multicellular organic structure is the most complex, most elusive, and most marvelous cosmic energy still mysterious to the intellect of modern man. The ancient Hindu writers called it "Maha-Shakti," the primordial life-energy, the cosmic force present in every fragment of the universe, from atoms to gigantic suns.

It is by far more complex than material energy and it works hidden from the objective sight of man. Every form of life, from the lowest to the highest, is a manifestation of a different spectrum of the bioenergy. Every variation in human beings, in their temperament, behavior, intellectual level, and other mental attributes springs from it. Personality changes that sometimes occur suddenly, often to the surprise of the individual concerned, are caused by it. Even the structure and the formation of the brain itself depend on the pattern of the bioenergy. Alterations in tastes, habits, and attitudes betoken changes in the *pranic* spectrum. In fact, the whole amazing complexity of life, the infinitely varied structures and forms, and the bewildering host of variations among human beings are all the effects of variation in the spectrum of this marvelous substance.

The law of heredity is operative because *prana* carries with it the hereditary characteristics ingrained in the spectrum. In dealing with mystical experience, genius, psi faculties, and insanity, we are concerned with variations in the composition of *prana,* or life-energy, and the study of this force will open up new vistas for mankind.

Somehow there is an impression among many people that human consciousness is a finally sealed and bound product with no possibilities of extension. In actual fact, consciousness in man is extremely flexible. Variation in intellect does not so much depend on variation in the brain as on the variation in consciousness. The span of consciousness in an individual depends on the quality of *prana* or pyschic energy, stimulating the brain and nervous system. The individual *prana* is drawn from the elements composing the body. The whole organism of a living creature is designed to produce a certain pattern of *prana,* which determines the nature of the consciousness exhibited by it, as also the structure of the personality displayed.

■ *This raises philosophical issues of great importance. Have we the least accurate knowledge of ourselves. Who am I? And what is this flame of consciousness that gives me awareness of myself and of the world around?*

The explanations furnished by great philosophers about this marvelous stuff we call life are the guesses of little children about the moon, mere fairy tales that appear absurd in the extreme at the very first glimpse of the Self.

Are we merely the ego-bound, small units of consciousness that think and act through the day and sink into oblivion of sleep during the night? To believe that this is all there is to it means discrediting the findings of modern psychology, which assert that we utilize only a small fraction of our mind and that the rest lies submerged as the unconscious.

If you agree with this view, then it is only one step further to acknowledge that the evolutionary process is a part of our unconscious. The true roots of our life do not lie in our body, in our brain, or our individual *prana*, but in the intelligent cosmic force or Universal *prana* that sweeps through the cosmos and is responsible for every organic structure of life. Whenever we think, imagine, or reason, we draw upon this cosmic reservoir of intelligent psychic power.

If this store of cosmic *prana* were inanimate, without a will and a direction of its own, we could very well flatter ourselves that every thought and fancy that we have is the product of our own volition. But since we are ourselves the products of this Superintelligent Cosmic Power, it would be illogical to the last degree to presume that our individual ideas and fancies are exclusively our own creations and have no relationship to the ocean of which we are but a tiny drop. When it is once admitted that mind and consciousness are cosmic entities, it would then be ridiculous to suppose that the thoughts and ideas in an individual atom of this Cosmic Consciousness can have an entirely independent existence and not reflect the will and design of the Cosmic Whole.

The knowledge of the mighty mechanism of *kundalini*, and of the expanded states of consciousness developed by it, brings us to the threshold of other momentous discoveries concerning life and mind. This stupendous nature of the world of consciousness that lies hidden from us in the normal state becomes at once perceptible. This leads to a reappraisal of the cosmos. In the light of the new experience of awakened *kundalini*, an immediate demand now arises, not only for the investigation of the colossal world of matter, which is perennially before our eyes, but also of the more complex, mysterious, and intriguing world of consciousness now unfolded before our inner sight. This perception of the hitherto completely unimaginable and unsuspected inner universe through the supersensory channel, developed by *kundalini*, is metaphorically known as the opening of the "Third Eye."

In ancient Hindu lore, Lord Shiva is said to be three-eyed because He is in possession of this supersensory channel of perception. An accomplished Yogi, who has raised *kundalini* from the base of the spine to the *sasha sara* in the head, is said in the ancient books to have attained to Shiva-consciousness. This implies the opening of the "Third Eye," by which the inner world of consciousness can be perceived.

■ *If it is demonstrated to the satisfaction of modern science that there is a physchophysiological mechanism in the human body responsible for mystical experience, genius, psychic gifts, and even insanity, doesn't this indicate then that the prophets and sages of the past were biologically gifted in a way that made lofty achievements possible?*

You are perfectly right. The barriers and conflicts between faith and faith, or creed and creed, are of our own making, and in fact the founders of religions and teachers of spirituality were simply more evolved human beings with no special privileges or concessions from the Creator, in spite of such claims made for them. The evolutionary mechanism in such individuals was active from birth or activated by some kind of discipline and way of life so that their brains were attuned to that transhuman state of consciousness that is the target of the evolutionary drive in the human race.

At the same time we have to bear in mind the important fact that the higher sphere of consciousness toward which mankind is slowly finding its way amidst vicissitudes, wars, and revolutions is of a more sublime and lofty nature than the average human consciousness, in the same way that the actual or professed adherence to high ethical standards of present human consciousness shows undisputed superiority over that of the beasts. Those who attained to the state of transhuman consciousness invariably demonstrated irrefutable evidence of lofty traits of character and conduct. The life stories of all well-known mystics, seers, and prophets are testimony to this fact. This is the target of the evolutionary process for us all, and the entire human race is evolving toward the state of being that we associate with the heavenly and the divine. There have been, and can be, no concessions and special privileges in a system of creation rooted in Law. We are all part of one evolutionary process.

■ *You say that this inner Self of the mystic projects itself in visions in concordance with his mental disposition. Do you mean that this inner Self possesses the power to materialize itself in the form of apparitions or lifelike visions?*

In order to answer this it is first necessary to define the limits of our mind. It is now generally recognized that by far the greater part of our conscious Self lives submerged below our outer personality. We are made aware of this subliminal part in dreams, hypnosis, sleepwalking, hysteria, or psychosis.

Taking dreams first, we find that sometimes they furnish us with solutions to problems that baffled us in waking life or recall to our memory events and incidents we had forgotten. Poets have received flashes of inspiration in dreams, scholars and thinkers hints for the solution of problems that had defied their waking skill or knowledge.

In hypnosis, the far more extended range of the subconscious mind is even more strikingly demonstrated. There is the incredible sense of time evinced by a subject, ordered in the hypnotic state to wake up after the expiry of a certain specific duration, or to act in a certain way—for instance, to open a book or move an object. Some hypnotic subjects are so precise in obeying a time command that they seem to be guided by an accurate chronometer. Feats of memory in hypnosis are no less remarkable. A skillful operator can evoke even embryonic memories, or the recollection of food taken, dress worn, work done, or persons met on a particular day, years earlier. These feats of memory are so convincing that it seems that not a single act out of millions performed in a lifetime is ever lost beyond recollection, but remains indelibly imprinted on the brain, ready to float to the surface when given appropriate stimulation.

Again, the subconscious mind also has the power to render the brain immune to pain. Hypnotism has been, and is still being used to induce anesthesia in major surgical operations. Mere suggestion creates immunity to agonizing pain for hours. We also know that suggestion administered during hypnosis can be used to cure even intractable diseases that had not been amenable to other treatment. The power of suggestion to cause vivid hallucinations in hypnotized subjects is really amazing. A blister or other pathological symptoms and reactions can be induced in the system merely by a suggestion in the trance state.

It is thus obvious that we use only a very small part of our consciousness and that it contains a vast reservoir of which we are not at all aware in our normal waking state. Psychologists have even gone so far as to suggest the existence of a collective unconscious in which even racial memories are stored. Instead of admitting straight away that mind has an independent existence and that the human or the animal brain is but an instrument through which it expresses itself, conditioned by individual characteristics, even psychologists evade the clear implications and resort to fantastic speculations and hypotheses to explain the extraordinary phenomena and extensive range of the subliminal self.

Such views will have to be revised in the light of the challenge by meticulously observed and conclusively proved psychic phenomena. And old theories and doctrines incompatible with the extrasensory functions of the mind will have to be discarded. Telepathy, mind reading, and prediction indisputably demonstrate the possibility of an individual mind to communicate with other minds without any intermediary material connecting link, startling facts that alone are sufficient to modify our present-day concepts about mind and matter. Even a single instance of foreknowledge that comes true in detail after the lapse of a certain period of time confronts us with an enigma that is insoluble on the basis of present-day theories about the universe.

It is therefore clear that our knowledge of ourselves is fragmentary and incomplete. Dissatisfied with the old answers and confronted by problems for which they have no solutions, many young scientists are now devoting their time and energy to exploration of the still imperfectly understood territory of mind and consciousness.

The mass of evidence collected is slowly tending to present a completely different picture of the mind than that drawn by the older philosophers and psychologists for whom the visible world of matter represented the sole reality of the universe. For our purpose, it is sufficient to point out here that the sphere of mind is a totally different proposition compared with the sphere of visible matter and its properties. Both ultimately owe their existence to one reality, at present inexplicable to our sense-bound intelligence. But for the purpose of relative study, it is useful to draw a distinction between the two. The energy that leads to sensation and thought and whose activity is manifested by electrical discharges in the brain and the nervous system, although

not perceptible to any of our restricted senses, might yet belong
to an altogether different category of natural forces than those
that are partially perceptible to us.

The moment we admit that mind and psychic energy can
belong to a class of cosmic energies of which we can have no
direct perception, because of the extremely narrow range of our
sensory equipment, we at once take up a more rational and more
realistic position than hitherto. The tendency to reduce creation
to the extremely restricted image that we perceive with our
sensory equipment has been one of the greatest obstacles in the
spiritual progress of mankind.

Even recent pronouncements of science about the ultimate
nature of matter have not tended to revise this fallacious view.
Were human beings to be deprived of two of their existing
senses and allowed to perceive the universe around them with
the help of the remaining three—say smell, touch, and taste only
—the whole creation would assume a totally different aspect.
When we assume that there can be other senses or channels of
perception at present unknown to us, it then becomes easy to
understand that one possessing such extra senses or channels of
perception would be able to perceive much more of the universe,
or at least those aspects of it which are totally imperceptible to
most of us, and of which we have no other means to apprehend.
For most people, such aspects of the universe become as if
nonexistent.

We consider a man to be dead when he fails to show symptoms invariably present in living organisms. Otherwise we have
no means of perceiving the existence of consciousness in a body
that is alive nor its absence in one that is dead. Mind and consciousness, as entities, are not perceptible to any of our normal
senses. Awareness is not merely a transient creation of our brains,
like the flame of a candle, which is extinguished when the candle
itself is consumed, but an eternal self-abiding stuff that has an

independent existence of its own, and the only way to account
for it is to treat it as something separate from the body, belonging to that class of created objects that are beyond the perceptual range of our senses.

We cannot treat consciousness as an evanescent stuff, appear-
ing and disappearing with the brain or the organic structure that
exhibits it, for the reason that in higher animals and man, consciousness assumes the colossal responsibility of reflecting and
interpreting the whole universe. A substance that mirrors the
universe and, in man, invests it with law and order, interpreting
it consistently to the minutest details, investigating and meas-
uring it from the invisible atoms to the stupendous stars, inter-
linking it with immeasurable spans of time and distance, cannot
be a by-product of biochemical processes without an independent status of its own. On the contrary, it should be palpably
apparent from even a cursory study that human consciousness,
as the fundamental stuff in terms of which we know, understand, and measure the cosmos, must be the basal substance,
born of the intelligence that we perceive working throughout the
universe.

It is incredible to what extent intellect can deceive itself with
its own sensory logic. The reality or permanency that we ascribe
to the cosmos is, in fact, a product of our own mind! Apart from
it, who can know or demonstrate what "reality" or "permanency" means? We ascribe reality to the visible universe but,
strange to say, deny it to the intangible stuff that is the origin of
the idea and the creator of the terms coined to express it, for-
getting that this very idea or concept could never arise did not
our own mind, in some mysterious way, partake of its nature
and were we not already familiar with it. From every point of
view, therefore, it is obvious that we have undervalued consciousness and failed to attach that importance to it that it deserves
as the final arbiter of all that we observe and discover in the

universe. This omission has been due in part to defective systems of philosophy, to the initial narrow-orbited views of science, and also to the parochial, self-condemning doctrines of faith.

Can any reasonable man in touch with modern advances in science have a rational or conscientious objection to the idea that consciousness itself is a self-existing cosmic stuff, beyond the range of our individual mind and senses in the same way that the consciousness of a human being is beyond the range of perception of his fellow beings? It is clear that by the action of an energy of which we have no parallel in the material universe, this mighty, self-existing, eternal stuff expresses itself through all the innumerable varieties of life on earth, through their brains and other equipment rather like the waves emanating from a radio or a television station that find expression through innumerable receivers and television sets.

We have hitherto failed to give due attention to our consciousness because at the beginning of the present era of science, a few thinkers and scientists—unaware of what the future would unfold and captivated by their own opinions—gave free rein to still unverified and unseasoned views about man, his soul and the beyond. Since these agnostic views still form the guidelines of most text books of science, philosophy, and psychology, modern students develop a bias for materialistic thought from the very commencement of their career. The result has been that apart from exceptionally healthy intellects that shake off the tentacles of materialism as the forerunners of morbid thought, many of the products of modern universities emerge entirely skeptical about the spiritual side of man. Consequently they have no hope in the perfection of humankind or the attainment of a more lofty and sublime level of human existence.

Starting from the premise of an ever-abiding, independent consciousness, it would be but rational to assume that the human soul, a marvelous invisible mirror that reflects the whole material cosmos, and at the same time is conscious of its own existence, is but a drop in a stupendous, all-pervading, deathless ocean of consciousness, interpenetrating the universe. But because of its extremely subtle and unconditioned nature, it is imperceptible to our senses and beyond all that we can know, classify, or understand by our mind and intellect. It is this entirely unfamiliar nature of consciousness, unlike anything else in our experience, that makes it extremely difficult for us to allot it its due position in the universe perceptible to our senses.

It is this unfamiliarity with the ground of our own being that makes *Samadhi*, or mystical experience, so overwhelming for the initiate. In the expanded state of consciousness the soul, for the first time, comes in direct contact with its substance and source, and in an instantaneous flash of recognition, realizing its own unconditioned and deathless nature, surpassing any former experience, soars to immeasurable heights of ecstasy and bliss. This is the reason for the unshakable conviction of immortality that pervaded the mind of every mystic and sage who had the supreme experience. In this condition, for the first time, the human mind comes into contact with other spheres of creation than the material universe it normally perceives.

In this light, a dispassionate assessment of the position should leave one in no doubt that the human consciousness, being a droplet of an inexhaustible and infinite ocean, can manifest itself in a more enlarged and potent way under certain circumstances. At the same time, it can also be inferred that this enlargement and increase in potency can be effected by a transformation of the brain and the sensory equipment, as has already happened in the organic kingdom during the march of evolution from the lowest to the highest states of its manifestation, culminating in man. Perhaps the most amazing omission in modern thinking has been that while thinkers avidly conceived the past, allowing their imagination to roam over a vista of thousands of millions of years, watching life climbing step by step from the primary organisms to anthropoids and man, they hardly cared to look ahead and estimate what would be the stature of future man if the organic impulse that raised him to his present estate continues its activities undiminished for another lengthy span of time.

■ *What is the final target of the evolutionary processes in man?*

The final target of the evolutionary processes is to carry the whole of mankind toward a higher dimension of consciousness. One significant lesson that we can draw from biology, from the innumerable forms of life inhabiting the earth, from minute cellular organisms to the mammals, is that not only are the physical forms of the various species and groups infinitely varied, but also there is a variation in the mental efficiency and instinctual responses of the various classes of creatures—in other words, variation in the state of consciousness. The performances of the dolphin appear amazing compared to other fishes, because of this difference in the degree of intelligence. Difference in intelligence also indicates difference in consciousness. This means that the whole gamut of organic life consists of an infinite variety in the patterns of consciousness of the various species and groups. We find this phenomenon clearly exhibited in human beings.

We see an endless variety in the degree of intelligence exhibited by members of the human race and can compare this gradation to the steps of a staircase leading from the bottom of a hill to its summit. Some categories of men stand virtually at the base of the hill and others on the top. The number of those who can be considered to have attained the summit—there are variations among these also—is extremely small. Most of the climbers are distributed on the intermediary steps. They are not all alike;

each one of them is in some respects different from his companions standing on the same rung. Let us suppose that the individuals at the top represent the highest intellectuals and the most talented men and women, who play outstanding roles in every field of intellectual and artistic activity and have always done so throughout the past. The point now arises whether these distinguished individuals at the top of the hill represent the last limit of human intelligence or whether there are still some heights even beyond.

Taking into account the enormous gulf intervening between a man of low intelligence and an intellectual prodigy—and the immense number of gradations between the two—would it not be unreasonable to suppose that the last limit represents the final boundary to which human intelligence can proceed?

A glance at the outstanding geniuses born during the historical period is sufficient to show that at no time was it possible to anticipate or foresee the stature of an exceptionally intelligent and versatile human being to be born in a subsequent epoch. Some of them outshone their predecessors to an amazing degree and were, in their turn, outshone by others to an extent that could not be anticipated. It would therefore be illogical to suppose that the highest talent of our day will not be outmatched to an unbelievable extent by the gifted mind of the future.

On the analogy of what has occurred in the past, the conclusion is irresistible that mankind will continue to produce specimens of extraordinary intelligence and talent so surprisingly superior to those we know that it would be extremely difficult, if not impossible, to form an accurate image of them in the light of our experience of the present or past.

The next question is whether this progression of human intellect will continue indefinitely in the ages ahead or whether it will come to an end at a certain limit. If the progression continues indefinitely it would be impossible to frame a correct picture of the highest geniuses that may adorn mankind in the course of the next few hundred years. If, however, there is to be a limit to the growth of intellect it would undoubtedly imply a cessation of progress, marking the zenith beyond which there would be either stagnation or decline. The continued progression in the past belies the supposition that there could be an end to this process in the foreseeable future.

What is of particular relevance to this theme is the fact that continued enhancement in the intellectual stature of genius necessarily implies continued progress of the race and the continued development of human potential, both mental and physical. Considering the fact that enhancement of intellect signifies increase in awareness, it would also mean that human consciousness will continue to show an occasional prodigious leap in dimension in the leading geniuses of the race. Such a conclusion is pregnant with tremendous implications.

In the first place it suggests that since the geniuses of an age represent the frontier of consciousness to which the race has progressed at that time, the mass of mankind will continue to show a progressive development in its intellectual endowment to keep pace with the enhancement in the stature of the geniuses. Secondly, that the continued improvement in the mental caliber of the men of genius will lead in the course of time to a height of intelligence and a state of consciousness quite beyond our present conception. Even now it is extremely difficult, if not impossible, for a man of average intelligence to form a correct image of the highly talented mind of a Plato, Shankaracharya, Omar Khayyám, Shakespeare, or an Einstein. This effort will be infinitely more difficult if we try to draw the picture of a future outstanding genius, towering head and shoulders above the highest specimens of the present or the past.

It is intriguing to ponder the issue whether, at any time in the development of the intellect, the talented man of the future will

come to the edge of what we can classify as human consciousness, and start to develop the rudiments of a new faculty that
transcends it; and that, like the mysterious processes occurring
in the brain of a lightning mathematical calculator or chess
prodigy, arrives at the solution of a problem without having
followed the complicated procedures that lead up to it.

We find fleeting glimpses of this faculty in almost every man
and woman at one time or the other. In our sudden likes
and dislikes of people, in the sudden assessment of bewildering
situations, in flashes of intuition concerning complicated busi-
ness propositions, in prophetic glimpses of the future, revelations
in dreams, and in numerous other matters in which we obtain
sudden insights into the reality without having recourse to reasoning, we actually stand at the parting of the ways where a new
faculty emerges in our own consciousness, arriving at conclusions
that the intellect would take considerable time to resolve. This
type of insight is often found to be particularly marked among
talented men in skilled professions, as for instance among physicians, lawyers, military commanders, psychologists, and the like.

It is well known that almost all outstanding men of genius
possess this faculty to a greater or lesser extent in relation to the
particular branch of knowledge in which they excel. Many great
poets and writers have clearly ascribed their compositions to a
spontaneous flow, absolutely independent of their own effort
and ideation. Hard work and deep absorption only help to develop it. Apart from geniuses, we also find this faculty operative
in the case of children who exhibit extraordinary talent in music,
painting, mathematics, invention, and the like at an extremely
young age, even before intellect has begun to function fully.

There is no explanation for these sudden flashes of insight or
sudden developments of precocious talents, sometimes even without education, unless we admit the existence of a dormant faculty
in the human brain that works more or less erratically and often

independently of the deliberate thought of a person. But even with all the vagueness and unpredictability attending this phenomenon, there can be no doubt about the fact that this intuitive sense has always played and still plays a decisive role in shaping and ordering the life of humanity, and that some of our most impulsive thoughts and acts owe their origin more to this intuitive faculty than to the deliberate calculations and conclusions of the intellect.

Judged in the light of the historical evidence already available, it is not difficult to infer that the human mind is evolving in a direction where a new channel of perception superior to the existing senses, and a new source of knowledge superior to the intellect, will adorn the consciousness of evolved human beings. The present investigation into extrasensory perception and psi phenomena will ultimately lead to the same conclusions that I am expressing here. That some individuals possess these faculties and that, broadly speaking, there is a basic similarity in their manifestations, is a clear indication that certain common psychic or biological factors are involved, pointing to one basis for all the phenomena. It is these extraordinary faculties—the essential attributes of a higher state of consciousness—that the ancient Indian treatises on Yoga and the occult have described as the *vibhutis*, or *siddhis*, or the opening of the "Third Eye."

■ *What is your view about the future of mankind?*

It is an inherent tendency of the human mind to build its image of the future on its experience of the present. In our own day we have seen the industrial revolution sweeping over the earth, flooding it with every kind of device to minimize the expenditure of human energy and to secure in every possible way protection from natural calamities, ensuring safety and comfort for the flesh. We can still safely count on technology to bring about yet undreamed-of revolutions in the mode of life and the environment of mankind. Fantastic achievements of science and technology in the future form the themes of science fiction books and provide material to imaginative writers for their sometimes unbelievable forecasts, but the real subject on which predictions about the future ought to be made is the condition of man himself.

The main issue that should receive the major share of our attention is whether physically, mentally, and morally man will continue to exist as he is now, or whether there will occur a change in this chief actor in the drama of the future. The fact that he may make fabulous progress in science and technology and be capable of even more prodigious feats of speed, engineering, mechanical skill, combative prowess, communication, and surgery is not enough to guarantee that man's own inner being and external behavior will change for the better in harmony with future great advances in knowledge.

Viewed in the light of the past, we see no noteworthy change for the better in the thinking and behavior of man in our times than at the end of the last century, or even before the birth of technology and science. The human world is still divided into segments, torn with dissension and hatred. It is still in the grip of nerve-shattering competition, perhaps more prey to tension, depression, anxiety, and worry than ever before.

In the more advanced nations, this lack of mental serenity and equilibrium is reflected in ruined peace of mind, disrupted family life, errant behavior, damaged marital relationships, and especially an alarming increase in neurotic and psychotic conditions of mind. If the present day—with all the convulsions and upheavals that are taking place—is treated as a sample of the state of humanity during the next few hundred years, were industry and technology to continue their progress with the same nerve-racking competition, interstate rivalry, armaments race, devastating wars, population explosions, air and water pollution, and the rest, then it should not be difficult for an imaginative person to picture the horrible state of the future individual and society as a whole and the dreadful effect it will have on the human mind. The reason why there is no stability and no limit to man's thinking and planning is because he himself is in a state of movement toward a destination still unknown to himself.

What my own experience has disclosed is that man is *not* evolving into a living computer with all the facts and figures of technology at his finger tips, with all the knowledge of the sciences on his tongue, but is slowly developing within himself a new pattern of consciousness, with a new channel of perception that, transcending intellect, will bring him in intimate contact with intelligent forces of Creation, expanding his mental horizon to an inconceivable extent, completely beyond the ablest thinkers of our time.

The human race is evolving toward a model that is completely different from any forecasts that can be made in our present conditioned state. We find it difficult to envisage a model of consciousness endowed with supersensory faculties, with power to penetrate into regions of life and mind entirely inaccessible to a normal man at the present time. That such channels of perception are possible we can readily infer from the fact that various specially gifted men and women throughout history have displayed some aspects of these faculties.

The intellect will remain intact, enhanced, augmented, and even more penetrating than at present. But what is of paramount importance in this evolutionary transformation of man is that every individual consciousness will be a pool of undiminishing happiness and bliss, aware of its own infinite and immortal nature, as one drop of an all-pervading infinite ocean of life.

This evolutionary goal of mankind is still hidden from the view of scholars and scientists as well as of ordinary men and women. It is as difficult for them to form even a mental picture of it as it is for a man of restricted intelligence to place himself in the position of a great intellectual. In the same way it is difficult for even the highest intellects of our time to frame a mental picture of the expanded consciousness that will be the precious heritage of future mankind.

Inside the gross tabernacle of human flesh there is slowly developing a radiant body of ethereal living light for the man and woman of the future. Many individuals of our day have occasional glimpses of this slowly developing luminous garment of the soul within—in vivid replendent dreams, in lustrous visionary experiences, in the perception of a luminous glow of brilliant flashes of light during meditation or other forms of spiritual exercise. Clothed in his vesture of light, the individual consciousness of the future will find itself surrounded by regions of everlasting glory and bliss, heralding its entry into the subtler levels of Creation. From this point, the world of consciousness will open its door wide for the future race to explore the most marvelous inner universe now opened to its sight.

■ *How can the average person achieve higher consciousness and help in the evolution of the race?*

The surest way should be to voluntarily develop the *characteristics* of higher consciousness. For instance, to always keep in mind that there is no barrier, no distinction, no wall between man and man. Whenever we see another person, though we may act in the normal way towards him, at the back of our minds should be the thought that the same consciousness, the same Divine substance, that is talking, hearing and listening in me, is also talking, hearing and listening in him; that it is one substance, one cosmic medium, that is expressing itself in all human beings.

This will be in accordance even with the saying of the Christ, "Treat thy neighbors as thyself." And it is also the teaching of the Bhagavad Gita, to treat all fellow human beings as your own self. This would be, perhaps, the most effective way to melt the barriers which are created by the ego—to always put oneself in the shoes of another.

Somehow, perhaps by the grace of God, I had this feeling from a very early age. It came as an urge. So even in my official capacity with the state government, if anybody came to me for consultation, I would wait for a few minutes, put myself in his place, and then give the advice. Even now I do it. It may be unpleasant or it may be pleasant, but I say to myself: "Now, how would I react if somebody were to give me false advice and waste my time and energy?" That is one of the main reasons why I keep so aloof from having disciples.

The time has come when, before giving intensive training to individuals, we *must* examine them both physically and mentally, because some minds are so delicately balanced that the least wrong advice can be disastrous for them. This frequently happens. Psychiatric clinics have many such cases, persons who are mentally unhinged because of concentration or some other occult practices.

This is also the reason why I think that every word I say should be tested. I would never like to see a single idea in my teachings that would mislead humanity or a section of it. So I am always cautious in my writings: Before accepting what I say, weigh it in the scale of your reason and test it in the crucible of your experience.

Another very powerful exercise is to keep before the mind's eye an image of Cosmic Consciousness. Or, if one believes in a God, to imagine that it is a Divine Consciousness, a presence, an immanence, an ethereal eye spread all over the universe—omniscient, omnipresent, and omnipotent.

The third would also be a corollary to the first: That since you now think—and you believe—that all men are yourself, having all the same feelings and emotions, and are also expressions of the same energy, you should act in ways that will help them, either by advice or by teaching, or by backing their prospects or by raising them up if they are fallen. Or by advising them where they are mistaken, trying to help them in the same way we would like to be helped when we are in distress. This would be an effective method.

A fourth exercise would be—in the morning and evening or at any convenient time—to sit in contemplation of Divinity, Cosmic Consciousness, God, Brahma, or by whatever name you call it, and continue thinking and meditating on it, reflecting on it as you would think, meditate or reflect on a very stubborn problem that needed to be solved. Try to build up the image in the mind, an image of an infinite extension, of an endless duration in time. And then dwell on these thoughts, and never allow the mind to become quiescent or to go into sleep. This exercise is given in many Yoga manuals.

The mind should remain alert, just as it remains alert when we are solving a problem, when we are concentrating on a mathematical proposition, or when we are studying a subject. We should keep the mind alert and reflect on the attributes of God—once, twice or thrice a day—in a devout mood, and offer this contemplation as a prayer to the Almighty to help us raise our consciousness.

The fifth would be to live a life in harmony with one's relatives, friends, and even strangers, in harmony with one's conscience and in harmony with the teachings of great religious prophets—not to be sanctimonious or prudish, but to have healthy instincts, to practice moderation and always to behave in a manner that is noble. High moral caliber goes side by side with an elevated state of consciousness, so all these disciplines are necessary, because the stage we are reaching for is composed of all these attributes. If we voluntarily cultivate them we help the evolutionary forces to build up the consciousness that will be the heritage of the future man.

■ *It is important, then, that the possibilities implicit in* kunda-lini *become widely known?*

Yes, with the Secret of *Kundalini* already known—but waiting to be accepted—the clinching proof for what I am disclosing can come any day, like a bolt from the blue. It will sweep away the resistance and lead to a cataclysmic upheaval in human thought seldom witnessed before.

Imagined in the context of the potentialities present in *kunda-lini* the vision of the future is so alluring, so full of beauty and majesty, so replete with astounding achievements and possibili-ties for the race, that it is not possible to draw even a distant image of it.

Suffice it to say that, in the congenial environment that will be created in the near future—as the result of evolutionary pressures exerted by racial consciousness and the growing knowledge of the evolutionary mechanism—a larger and still larger number of spiritual geniuses will be born in all parts of the world to aid the leaders in every field of human endeavor.

They will build a tension-free, harmonious world in which everyone is provided with the basic needs and has an equal op-portunity to perfect himself.

The constant state of crisis and desperation—with diplomats

running here and there frantically to extinguish nascent fires—
is a strongly marked feature of the world today. Such unavoidable
tense anxiety states are fatal for the evolutionary growth of the
human brain. In such an atmosphere, with the transformative
processes resistlessly working in the human body, the result can
only be escapism or perversion and distortion of the growing
mind.

Those who believe that this can be controlled or remedied are,
to put it frankly, living in a paradise of fools. It will progressively
deteriorate, unless the evolutionary needs are met. It is a symptom of a growing mental distemper.

The earth is to become an abode of a graceful, highly intelligent cosmic conscious race. Wafted to another dimension of
mind, as the result of organic changes in the brain, it will be
equally cognizant of both the worlds—the outer and the inner
or the material and the spiritual.

It will be brought in touch with another level of creation, other
intelligences and states of being pervading the universe, a universe now completely shut out from our sight because of the
limited capacity of our brains.

It is not some aliens from other planets but we who will be
the future enlightened denizens of the earth, just as we have
been of the savage past. The life of our distant progeny will be
so full of charm and beauty, harmony and music, love and ro-
mance, adventure and exploit in space (both inner and outer),
wonders and marvels, that no imaginative thinker has so far been
able to frame a picture of it.

They will have such an extended span of life, long-lasting
youth and vigor, freedom from illness, want and oppression, that
this will be the Kingdom of God, Paradise, or Nirvana, prophe-
sied by the great seers and prophets of the past. It is to be gained,
not in a hypothetical heaven, but here on earth, in the organic

frame of man. It is the sublime state of beatitude that is promised in every holy scripture of mankind.

In this vision of the future, even the ideas of "Resurrection,"
"Liberation" and "Salvation" will find fulfillment in a dramatic
way. What we now experience or know of as clairvoyance, astral
projection, telepathy, premonition or prophesy, are but faint
glimpses of a future enormously-extended state of consciousness.

In rapport with the ocean of Cosmic Intelligence, man will be
able to trace the whole drama of life on earth, and even on other
orbs, and know himself for what he really is—a drop in the everlasting universal ocean of Being. He will be eternally serene and
unaffected by the costumes he wore and the scenes in which he
acted in all the aeonic dramas since life started on this planet.

Therefore, whether he awakens to his majesty now or in his
still-distant future progeny, the enlightened individual will realize
himself as the Sun that had merely lit up the stage. He will see
the scenario and the action of the dramas that he thought he had
played—whether as a sub-human or a civilized human being—
but will himself remain untouched and unchanged, to come out
of the happy or unpleasant episodes as a sleeper wakens from a
dream.

About the Author

Gopi Krishna was born in 1903 to parents of Kashmiri Brahmin extraction. His birthplace was a small village about twenty miles from the city of Srinagar, the summer capital of the Jammu and Kashmir State in northern India. He spent the first eleven years of his life growing up in this beautiful Himalayan valley.

In 1914, his family moved to the city of Lahore in the Punjab which, at that time, was a part of British India. Gopi Krishna passed the next nine years completing his public school education. Illness forced him to leave the torrid plains of the Punjab and he returned to the cooler climate of the Kashmir Valley. During the succeeding years, he secured a post in the Public Works Department of the state, married and raised a family.

In 1946 he founded a social organization and with the help of a few friends tried to bring about reforms in some of the outmoded customs of his people. Their goals included the abolition of the dowry system, which subjected the families of brides to severe and even ruinous financial obligations, and the strictures against the remarriage of widows. After a few years, Gopi Krishna was granted premature retirement from his position in the government and devoted himself almost exclusively to service work in the community.

In 1967, he published his first major book in India, *Kundalini — The Evolutionary Energy in Man.* Shortly thereafter it was published in Great Britain and the United States and has since appeared in eleven major languages. The book presented to the Western world for the first time a clear and concise autobiographical account of the phenomenon of the awakening of Kundalini, which he had experienced in 1937. This work, and the sixteen other published books by Gopi Krishna have generated a steadily growing interest in the subjects of consciousness and the evolution of the brain. He also travelled extensively in Europe and North America, energetically presenting his theories to scientists, scholars, researchers and others.

Gopi Krishna's experiences led him to hypothesize that there is a biological mechanism in the human body which is responsible for creativity, genius, psychic abilities, religious and mystical experiences, as well as aberrant mental states. He asserted that ignorance of the working of this evolutionary mechanism was the main reason for the present dangerous state of world affairs. He called for a full scientific investigation of his hypothesis and believed that such an objective analysis would uncover the secrets of human evolution. It is this knowledge, he believed, that would give mankind the means to progress in peace and harmony.

Gopi Krishna passed away in July 1984 of a severe lung infection and is survived by his wife, three children and grandchildren. The work that he began is currently being carried forward through the efforts of a number of affiliated foundations, organizations and individuals around the world.

OTHER BOOKS BY GOPI KRISHNA